THE PHILOSOPHY OF VIAGRA

VALUE INQUIRY BOOK SERIES

VIBS

Volume 230

a volume in
Philosophy of Sex and Love
PSL
Adrianne McEvoy, Editor

THE PHILOSOPHY OF VIAGRA

Bioethical Responses to the Viagrification of the Modern World

Edited by
Thorsten Botz-Bornstein

Rodopi

Amsterdam - New York, NY 2011

Cover Photo: www.dreamstime.com

Cover Design: Studio Pollmann

The paper on which this book is printed meets the requirements of "ISO 9706:1994, Information and documentation - Paper for documents - Requirements for permanence".

ISBN: 978-90-420-3336-8
E-Book ISBN: 978-94-012-0036-3

Printed in the Netherlands

CONTENTS

Introduction

VIAGRA, LIFESTYLE, AND THE PHILOSOPHICAL PERSPECTIVE

Thorsten Botz-Bornstein

1. A New Lifestyle Drug

The impotency remedy Viagra is the "fastest selling drug in history" (McGinn, 1998, p. 44). It is no longer a medical phenomenon, but also a cultural icon, appearing in television sitcoms as a pretext for jokes or as a murder weapon, rivaling with "Coca-Cola as one of the most widely known brands in the world" (*New York Times*, 21 August 2003). Viagra (as well as similar products like Levitra and Cialis) has socio-cultural implications not limited to sexuality, but concerns various parts of our cultural landscape. The fact that popular culture embraced Viagra with such an enthusiasm is due to a paradox: though Viagra has been established on the assumption that impotency is a purely medical (and not social or psychological) phenomenon, the drug can also be used for recreational purposes, that is, within socially and psychologically established contexts. The cultural status of Viagra becomes even more complex as the borderlines between recreational and non-recreational sex are blurred.

In spite of, or because of, the narrow humanistic basis offered by its producers, Viagra has attained status as a lifestyle drug and men between the ages of 18 and 45 are the fastest growing consumer group. In principle, the term lifestyle drug encompasses "drugs that fulfill non-medical or non-health-related outcomes" (Rubin & Wylie, 2009, p. 57). However, in the modern world, when something is addressed as a "life-style drug," the formulation very often includes a self-sufficient moral justification that can be challenged only with much difficulty.

Being relatively convincing in terms of bio-medical efficiency, critical discussions of Viagra have so far mainly been developed by – apart from Christian blogs evaluating the drug's use for either procreative or recreational purposes – the (often feminist) "Liberal Arts" camp where Pfizer (the maker of Viagra) is reproached for its profit-oriented negation of any psychological, social, emotional, or relational components involved in impotency. Here one addresses the fact that Viagra reduces a holistic masculine problem "to only six inches (or so) of a man's body" (Plante, 2006, p. 379). Or one criticizes that Viagra sexuality is construed from a male point of view, which ignores the distinctiveness of female sexuality. Criticism ridicules Viagra's mechanical imagery of a "techno-fix" (Vares & Braun, 2006), not only intensifying the medicalization of impotency current since the early 1980s, but also making "sex into a medical function like digestion" (Tiefer, 2003, p. 2). Viagra renders masculinity as a mere problem of chemical engineering, plumbing, and hydraulics. A further concern is that through Viagra, the traditional gender role of the "potent man and the happy woman" is restored without any critical revision (Loe, 2004, p. 21).

Ironically, as long as it declares psychological, social, emotional, and relational components to be the monopoly of women, feminist discourse is responsible for a reductionist sexuality. "Woman's sexual lives are contextualized," writes Leonore Tiefer because their sexual experiences depend more on "social context (relationship, cultural background, past sexual experiences)" than on genital functioning (Tiefer, 2003, p. 2). It would be better to postulate such standards for sexual behavior in an ungendered fashion.

While Viagra has changed the sex-life in industrialized countries, it is interesting to note that these changes did not come along as waves of a sexual revolution similar to what the industrialized world experienced in the 1970s, telling us that our sexual mores are too narrow, that we should liberate ourselves from taboos and social constraints. Viagra is the drug of a consumer society that has little time to reflect upon fundamental issues. As it stands, Viagra appears as the drug of a capitalist society convinced that any efficient medication approved by the state signifies progress and higher levels of happiness. It is therefore remarkably compatible with bourgeois lifestyle. Strangely, the few items that might strike us as provocative (such as embarrassing television ads) are quickly passed over. Contrary to what was the norm in the provocative 1970s, anything today that is potentially obscene is hastily stifled under a veil of utter normalcy.

I say "strangely" because, paradoxically, the existence of Viagra owes so much to the culture of sexual liberation. Viagra values individualism and self-improvement as well as the eschewal of external authority except for the scientific one. Other preconditions for the successful implementation of Viagra have been established through a more hidden agenda. One of the "side effects" of sexual liberation is that it brought about a sense of competitiveness in the realm of sexuality that would have been unthinkable in earlier decades. These changes seem to have made Viagra more necessary than ever. Allan Bloom speaks out as somebody who knows what sexuality was like in the 1950s:

> In the past a man could think he was doing a wonderful thing for a woman, and expect to be admired for what he brought. But that was before he could be pretty sure that he was being compared and judged, which is daunting. (…) It is easier for men to get gratification than it used to be (…). But at least some of these advantages for men are offset by nervousness about their sexual performance. (Bloom, 1987, p. 124)

While uncritical Viagra discourses seem to flow directly out of a culture that rationalizes and technicizes everything including sexuality, there is a paradox that lets Viagra-enhanced sexuality stand out as a peculiar social phenomenon. While, on the one hand, sexuality is reduced to hydraulics and chemistry, on the other hand, large efforts are made to extend the scope of Viagra beyond the limits of the bedroom, granting male potency a quasi mythical status. For the most part, what is in question is not just sexual pleasure, but also old myths of male dominance applied to fields ranging from professionalism to creativity. Elie Metchnikoff, a forerunner in techno-fix methods, insisted that sexual activity is connected to poetic genius (Marshall & Katz, 2002, p. 51). This means that the recent terminological shift from "impotency" to "erectile dysfunction" is only cosmetic. In reality, the "plumbing problem" is still perceived as a character flaw and "fixing" the problem could transform a man's life.

2. Viagra and Philosophy

Lafontaine reminds us that not only Viagra, but also impotence is a phenomenon engendered by civilization because, under natural conditions, very few individuals could reach or outlive the age of reproduction (Lafontaine, 2009, p. 61). It seems that, at the culminating point of this development of civilization, Viagra has become the symbol of modernity concentrating in itself a sort of achieved utopia in which everything promptly materializes if we only manage to exclude existential complications from our lives. According to Raymond Aron, the perfect state of modernity is characterized by "the cult of success, individual initiative, violence of competition, optimism about the future and rejection of existential anguish, reducing of every situation to technically soluble problems" (Aron, 2001, p. 297). In the realm of sexuality, our age is not the age of tragic eroticism, but rather that of linear enhancement, as Allan Bloom has noted right after the sexual revolution: "The eroticism of our students is lame. It is not the divine madness Socrates praised; or the enticing awareness of incompleteness and the quest to overcome it" (Bloom 1987, p. 132). Were Bloom living today, he could state how Viagra has eliminated more thoroughly than ever things like passion, hope, despair, and "a sense of the twinship of love and death" (p. 123).

All this shows that Viagra needs to be examined not only from a sociological, but also from a philosophical point of view. Sociology mainly studies how the social status of the drug interacts with certain situational aspects. A philosophical discussion of Viagra should reach beyond utilitarian considerations, beyond benefits and burdens. With Viagra, we are confronted with a powerful rationalization of sexuality to which philosophy can pose an "erotic rationality" derived from its own tradition. Major philosophers like Spinoza, Schopenhauer, and Kierkegaard, and, in the twentieth century, Sartre, Merleau-Ponty, Levinas, Deleuze, Foucault, Alexandre Kojève, Allan Bloom and Luce Irigaray – to name only some – have been interested in exploring sexuality from points of view uninfluenced by theories constructed by scientists.

Since Plato, philosophy has known that scientific explanations, which claim to give an exhaustive account of erotic perception, are misleading. At the earliest stage of Western philosophy love was seen as a paradoxical form of rationality/irrationality. Two thousand years later, philosophy has not entirely forgotten this heritage. The philosopher James Waddell urges us to find "tools that are forged in the heat of erotic passion as it is lived to help us spot nonsense and to make sense of our own experience" (1997, p. 2); and Sophie Bourgault suggests in the present volume that philosophy should be seen as a "Viagra of the soul." Inspiring is the particularly paradoxical nature of Eros, which represents both a form of Platonic rationality *and* an irrational, irreducible quality that can be used as a critical tool able to debunk various forms of scientific rationalizations of sexuality – one of which is the clinical-sexological discourse on Viagra.

Some hold that philosophy has already lost too much of its erotic heritage and that it is no easy task to reinstall philosophy as a profoundly erotic cure. Jean-Luc Marion deplores the idea that

> philosophy has lost even the desire for love; indeed, sometimes one would almost believe that philosophy hates love. Philosophy does not love love, which reminds her of her origin and her dignity, her powerlessness and her divorce. She therefore silently ignores it, when she does not hate it throughout. (Marion, 2007, p. 3)

The present studies on Viagra try to bring philosophy back onto the classical track of eroticism. So far, there are very few serious philosophical attempts at tackling the Viagra phenomenon. Examples are "Deleuze on Viagra" by Annie Potts and Leonore Tiefer's "Doing the Viagra Tango" published in *Radical Philosophy*. The part of Viagra criticism that turns around technobody and cyborg studies comes probably closest to philosophical thought. Also worth mentioning is Vincent Del Casino's attempt to develop a "flaccid theory" as a form of weak theory that works against the logics of hardness, which "validates the flaccid, suggesting that we need not be hard to be active sexual (or social scientific) beings: there are multiple ways (for men) to practice sex that need not include an erection" (Del Casino, 2007, p. 911).

The present volume fills in a gap that has, so far, been yawning in the academic landscape. All contributors to this book are academic philosophers. Though all authors also use the most recent *scientific* literature on the subject, their philosophical interpretations of the Viagra phenomenon attempt to contradict and deconstruct a scientific vision of Viagra as the enhancer of self-esteem and sexual confidence based on the "hard facts" of scientific findings. Like other academic disciplines (sociology, anthropology, psychology, etc.) philosophers oppose narrow biologistic principles. However, the alternative they propose is a phenomenological, existentialist vision of erotic experience, sometimes connected to a criticism of modern society or simply of modernity as such.

Addressing Viagra from a philosophical angle is like viewing a phenomenon that has become very much embedded in our culture from a completely different perspective. The approach functions much like that of intercultural philosophy. What would the ancient Greeks or any thinker from another époque have said about Viagra? The results of many of the articles contained in the present volume come amazingly close to cross-cultural examinations of Viagra.

It is worth mentioning one of the few existing cross-cultural analyses of Viagra undertaken by Everett Yuehong Zhang in 2007. Zhang's work was sparked by the fact that the sales of Viagra in China were in sharp contrast to the high expectations of Pfizer. Zhang states that in China, the readiness to use the drug has clearly been compromised by Daoist principles internalized by Chinese consumers. Chinese medical classics as well as Daoist scriptures see

> impotence as a result of the loss of the *yin-yang* balance of *qi* in different locations, of an excessive loss of *jing*, or of the clogging of *qi*, and so on. These symptoms are all signs of a decline of vitality. This stands in stark contrast to the etiology of impotence as set out in biomedicine. (Zhang, 2007, p. 86 note 8).

The Chinese patient, an apparently simple peasant, was not convinced when his doctor explained to him a basic principle of Western biomedicine: "What does it mean to be potent? So long as you can do it each time with the help of Viagra, you are not impotent. You are potent" (p. 62). Zhang explains that traditional Chinese ethics of sexuality is "more concerned with the cultivation of life, or *overall* potency, and, as such, is in conflict with a globalized sexual ethics that focuses solely on reproduction and sexual pleasure" (p. 63). Chinese patients are most concerned with the threat that in the future they will be dependent on Viagra. This possibility is not sufficiently discussed in Western literature, in spite of findings highlighting the fact that "normal adults and adolescents taking Viagra regularly have problems with sexual relationships if they stop taking the drug" (Morales et al, 2005, quoted from Rubin 2009, p. 58). Similar observations have been made in Japan by Genaro Castro-Vázquez: a young man used to be happy with his initial Viagra prescriptions, but would become anxious later, believing that he had to take Viagra forever. The doctor explained to him that "if you are able to develop self-confidence you should be able to stop using Viagra," which resulted in the patient wearing a Viagra pill as an amulet (Castro-Vázquez, 2006, p. 123).

Many classical Greek philosophers have taken a view of sexuality similar to the aforementioned Chinese, presenting challenges to the narrow hedonism of Western societies. Stoicism for example, suggested that we simply disregard all those things that are not within our power. And Epicurus, in his Letter to Menoeceus, urges us to adopt a "sober reasoning" and to understand "that death is nothing to us but makes the mortality of life enjoyable, not by adding to life an unlimited time, but by taking away the yearning after immortality" (Epicurus, 1966, p. 98).

Consequently, many of the chapters in the present volume revolve around the classical themes of immortality and hedonism. The first four chapters represent attempts to view Viagra through the lenses of classical philosophy. Sophie Bourgault discusses Plato's Cephalus, who boasts about his erectile difficulties because he believes that "thanks to the death of his sex drive, he has grown increasingly appreciative of the pleasures of philosophy." Though this must seem strange for us today, Plato holds that too much physical health is not desirable and that disproportionate care for the body can be detrimental to the cultivation of virtue. Robert Vuckovich examines how Diogenes of Sinope, who lived with the fewest possessions and desires, would have responded to Viagra. Would he have found it unnatural if men want to do what comes naturally? Or would he have found men's dependency on this need for sexual satisfaction a form of enslavement to their passions? Would a cynic not hold, as Thomas Kapper contends, that men conspire through Viagra to prolong adolescence to the point of absolute absurdity? Kapper interprets Viagra in the light of Aristotle's *eudaimonia* as well as in the context of Stoic philosophy, which holds that the best-lived life is one that is in harmony with what occurs by nature. Kevin Guilfoy sees Viagra as an inverted value system of everything an older and wiser, but less virile St. Augustine would have appreciated. Similar to Diogenes, St. Augustine held that low libido or diminished sex drive leaves him at liberty to pursue knowledge and spiritual development. St. Augustine seems to be of particular interest for Viagra studies. Slavoij Žižek, in *The Ticklish Subject*, points to St. Augustine's interpretation of erectile difficulties as the Divine punishment for man's desire to become master of the universe (Žižek, 1999, p. 384). St. Augustine's philosophy is also of interest to Robert Redeker, who, in the present volume, contrasts the utopia created by Viagra with Augustine's transcendental utopia described in *The City of God.* Redeker shows that Campanella's utopia required love to become automatized and mechanized and that sex must be carried out at certain hours that were decided by the authorities beforehand. For Redeker this anticipates a major trait of Viagra in political philosophy.

Connie Price offers a critical survey of the academic and industrial machine known as the biosciences and discovers that "an ethical encounter with the issues of Viagra demonstrates the conservatism of bioethics as it has been defined for some forty years." In my own article on Viagra and Virtual Reality I show that, while Freud materialized desire and turned it into a sexual drive, Viagra dematerializes desire and turns it into a virtual quality. Anthony Okeregbe reflects Viagra against the Africanist perspective which views sexual virility primarily as the means of transmitting life. Okeregbe points out that the traditional African considers sex a sacred activity: "The sexual act, tied to the totality of human sexuality, is viewed as sacred because its value does not lie in the act itself." Interestingly, the popularity accorded Viagra in the West has rekindled confidence in herbal and traditional medicine in Africa and an herbal remedy known as the 'African Viagra' can now be bought online. Okeregbe is also intrigued by the fact that the Church has not condemned the use of Viagra. Dónal O'Mathúna questions the fact that "where human trials and tribulations have failed to succumb to religion, superstition, social engineering, (...) biomedical and pharmaceutical progress has won the day." He explains why solutions can still be found in "religious, philosophical and personal discussions that have characterized how people deal with suffering, illness, and death."

Claude-Raphaël Samama provides important psychoanalytical input, attacking clinical sexology in the most explicit fashion by confronting it with psycho-philosophical realities. Samama draws special attention to Lacan who, for the first time, put the decisive distinction between penis and phallus in a philosophical context. Samama is eager to establish desire as a *spiritual* process and shows that human sexuality cannot be linked to a periodical or instinctual physical "mechanics." This adds to the view developed by Okeregbe – though in a completely different context – that sex should always be seen as a vitalistic activity in the sense of a union of life-forms "requiring animalist capacity or what Aristotle calls soul-function."

In my own chapter on Viagra and American culture, I examine relationships between sexuality and race, echoing Okeregbe's statement that "nowhere is this valorization of the penis more evident than in the racialized black male sexuality portended by ancient texts, Victorian literatures, historical and autobiographical works as well as experiences from the slave trade." Through Viagra, sexual virility is put at the center of sexual culture, but it resides there not as a real quality but as a possibility, a purely potential quality or a sexual one-drop rule. The "one drop" can be considered a "racial Viagra."

Towards the end of the book, Herb Roseman approaches Viagra from a different angle and summarizes the history of the science of impotence in the light of T.S. Kuhn's model of scientific paradigms. He explains the particular position of Viagra within this development. Roseman also evaluates the utilitarian perspective provided by Mill and other philosophers and tries to understand how they would have reacted to the phenomenon of Viagra.

Roman Meinhold draws our attention to another paradigm, that of Arnold Gehlen's development of culture through the deficient nature of humanity. Meinhold attempts to view Viagra through this pattern, comparing it with the telescope or the night-vision apparatus. Meinhold investigates how Viagra marketing utilizes the drive of humans to improve themselves and their environment by at the same time comparing their own condition or status quo with those of others or with potential conditions. In a brief note, Roseman picks up the theme of natural selection and discusses Viagra in the context of Darwinism.

Finally, Bassam Romaya examines a series of interrelated social and cultural factors in the context of multifaceted, nationalist expectations of group productivity and the likelihood for reproduction, which ultimately privileges the lives of male-born erections over a subpopulation with alternative erections, or transerections.

One

EROS, VIAGRA, AND THE GOOD LIFE: REFLECTIONS ON CEPHALUS AND PLATONIC MODERATION

Sophie Bourgault

"Every man must honor Love [ἔρως]"
- Plato, *Symposium* 212b[1]

1. Introduction

It is well known that Plato's *Republic* is a conversation about justice and the good life. But what is often overlooked is that this conversation is initiated by a brief but significant exchange about aging and sexual impotence. At the very beginning of the *Republic*, when Socrates is welcomed into the house of the old metic Cephalus, the latter chooses to offer his greetings precisely by invoking his impotence. Far from feeling any shame at his erectile difficulties, the rich Cephalus in fact boasts about them. He believes that thanks to the death of his sex drive, he has grown increasingly appreciative of the pleasures of philosophy (328d). Cephalus prides himself on being radically different from his old friends, who all resent their impotence and equate the end of their sex lives with the end of life itself (a claim which invalidates the point often made by scholars to the effect that impotence was, until recently, something that was accepted with grace).[2]

> "When we meet," Cephalus says, "the majority complain about the lost pleasures they remember from their youth, those of sex, drinking parties, feasts, and the other things that go along with them, and they get angry as if they had been deprived of important things and had lived well then but are now hardly living at all." (*Republic* 329d)

Cephalus claims that he is much wiser about what living well entails; he contends that the release from sexuality has been a source of liberty and a great opportunity: "old age brings peace and freedom (…). When the appetites relax and cease to importune us (…) we escape from many mad masters" (329c). Thanks to the release from these 'mad masters' and more generally, to his moderate character, Cephalus believes he possesses what it takes to age well and to carry on a lengthy philosophical exchange.

But what the unfolding of the dialogue quickly reveals is that all this boasting is a mere charade: the conversation has only begun that Cephalus decides to leave the room, invoking the need to attend to a religious sacrifice. (331d) Now, the speedy departure of Cephalus has been variously interpreted, with some insisting that Cephalus had to leave on account of his advanced age (Cicero, 1956, p. 315; Javet, 1982, p. 244), of his democratic sympathies (Steinberger 1996) and on account of the fact that he represents the ancestral Athenian order, an order that ought to questioned by philosophy (Strauss, 1964; Bloom, 1968). Other scholars have suggested that it makes perfect sense for the impotent metic to eschew the conversation, since he would have had little to gain from it. According to C.D.C. Reeve for instance, "Cephalus cannot benefit from the elenchus because his character is already as good as Socrates'" (1988, p. 5). Reeve is not alone in suggesting that Cephalus is quite an honorable and moderate man: Stanley Rosen (2005, p. 26)[3] and Johannes Kakridis (1948, p. 39) also espouse such a reading. Contrary to this view, I will argue below that Cephalus does not possess the virtue of moderation and that he is not genuinely reconciled with his impending death and accompanying sexual impotence. Despite his own claim to the contrary, Cephalus would have been the first to rush to his doctor to ask for a prescription of Viagra if the blue pill had existed in Ancient Athens. *And what if he had done so*? What would have been Socrates' reaction if, instead of invoking religious duties in order to legitimize his withdrawal from the conversation, Cephalus had claimed that he needed to visit his doctor in order to get some Viagra? What would the following exchange have entailed?

The purpose of this paper is to carry out this thought experiment, in order to make the following set of claims. First, I want to argue that while Socrates would *not* have stopped Cephalus from visiting his doctor (for one thing, Socrates is no strict ascetic), he nevertheless would not have let him go without first offering the old man a few pieces of friendly advice regarding health and good patient-doctor relationships. Drawing on Plato's *Laws* and the *Charmides*, the first two parts of this paper will discuss these Platonic insights and indicate their remarkable timeliness. I will show that more than two thousand years before sociologists, sexologists and various critics of the pharmaceutical industry penned critical pieces about the "Viagra phenomenon" and lifestyle drugs, Plato offered sensible advice regarding hasty drug prescriptions and the need to consider the physiological and the psychological in tandem. I will also indicate that in Plato, the medical and the ethico-political rarely part ways and that each heavily informs the other. The quest for justice and moderation (*sophrosyne*) cannot be severed from the quest for health. Indeed, Thierry Ménissier was certainly right to depict Plato's *Republic* as "a great book on sickness" (1995, p. 356; translation mine).

After our discussion of disease, health and good doctors, I propose to turn to Plato's views regarding *eros* and moderation (*sophrosyne*). My goals here are twofold: I will first defend the claim (made briefly above) that Cephalus lacks true moderation, and I will briefly assess the significance of this moral deficiency. Second, I wish to argue that what the old man is in urgent need of, from a Platonic perspective, is not the cure provided by a little blue pill, but rather, that provided by the Viagra of the soul, philosophy—a profoundly *erotic* cure. Indeed, if Plato's work puts *eros* on trial, it also redeems it.

2. Prescriptions, Persuasion, and the Giving of Accounts

Plato's dialogues are peppered with analogies between the art of politics and the art of medicine: justice is said to be akin to health, and both are said to require much care, expertise, and love—a love meant to create concord and harmony in the body, the soul and the city (e.g. *Republic* 341a-342e; *Gorgias* 501a-505b).[4] In the *Symposium* for instance, Plato writes that: "A good practitioner knows how to affect the body and how to transform its desires (...) [his] task is to effect a reconciliation and establish mutual love between the most basic bodily elements. Medicine, therefore, is guided everywhere by the god of Love." (*Symposium* 186e-187a) In the *Laws*, it is in the context of exploring the similarities between good ruling and good medical practice that Plato offers us (through the mouth of his Athenian Stranger) one of his most sustained accounts of the good doctor (720a-721a). It is an account that warrants our attention for a moment, for it is this account that would have informed Socrates' judgment had he tried to counsel Cephalus before letting him run off to his doctor.

In the *Laws*, we learn that one of the most important traits that define a good physician according to Plato is that he (or she)[5] never rushes into giving a patient a 'prescription'—whether it is one that proposes the use of medication, of an incantation, or a particular change in diet (720c-d). Plato is not only convinced that most illnesses should be left to run their course (*Timaeus* 89a-d) but more significantly, that a 'prescription' should never be given by a doctor without first having had an extensive discussion with the patient. As the Athenian Stranger explains, the good doctor will patiently build "an empirical case-history by consulting the invalid and his friends; in this way he himself learns something from the sick and at the same time he gives the individual patient all the instruction he can" (*Laws* 720d). Ideally, the patient must be led to understand for him or herself why the 'cure' or diet to be adopted is sensible—which requires a lengthy exchange and detailed arguments. Persuasion is the name of the game, not compulsion. By contrast, a bad doctor "simply prescribes what he thinks best in the light of experience, as if he had precise knowledge, *and with the self-confidence of a dictator*. Then he dashes off on his way to the next slave-patient (...)" (*Laws* 720c; my italics). Socrates would thus likely have warned Cephalus to be suspicious of doctors who prescribe hurriedly and with assertive authority—a timely piece of advice given the speed with which doctors prescribe 'lifestyle' medications today and the great deference medical experts are the object of (Marshall, 2002). While Plato acknowledges that medicine is an art that requires extensive expertise, the proper position a patient should adopt vis-à-vis his doctor ought not to be one of blind submission but rather, one of willful, *informed* consent.

Part of what all this would mean, in contemporary terms, is that a sensible doctor would refuse to write hastily a prescription for a patient who merely seeks sexual 'enhancement', insisting on first having a lengthy discussion about the patient's needs, motivations, and entire way of living. More specifically, a good Platonic doctor would try to make the enhancement-seeker realize why his hedonist perspective on life might be in need of questioning. This is not to claim that (sexual) pleasure in itself ought to be repressed because it is 'bad' according to Plato. As Michel Foucault (1984) has convincingly shown, sexuality in ancient Greece was not principally informed by notions of 'good' and 'bad', of 'allowed' and 'forbidden'—and this observation certainly applies to Plato's way of approaching sexuality. As we will discuss further below, Plato does not empty human existence of intense pleasure nor does he seek to impose a repressive moral code on all erotic encounters.[6] But Plato is definitely interested in challenging the hedonist mottos that "more is better" and "bigger is better"—slogans that Plato puts in the mouth of Thrasymachus and Callicles[7] (two ballsy individuals equipped with souls Socrates desperately wishes to reform). In Socrates' view, Thrasymachus and Callicles have both failed to reflect on why not *any* kind of pleasure can be equated with the good life and why *pleonexia* (greed) ultimately comes down to tyranny.

Unsurprisingly, given his outlook on an unreflective type of hedonism, Plato believes that medicine ought not to be judged on the basis of how much pleasure it brings to human beings, but rather, on whether it leads to "what is best" (*Gorgias* 465a). Put differently, it is our minds—and not our genitals—that are to judge what constitutes a judicious usage of medicine and medication. The good doctor will not only take the time needed to have a proper discussion and avoid hasty prescriptions; she will also be proficient in the giving of accounts—accounts of what the nature of health is and, more specifically, what health of the body and health of the soul are all about (*Laws* 720c; cf. *Gorgias* 501b). Plato undoubtedly puts high demands on doctors: not only should they have a solid knowledge of how to treat the body; they should also understand how the latter relates to the human mind. After all, each deeply affects the other, as Plato insists throughout his work, but particularly in the *Timaeus*.

It is largely on the basis of the *Timaeus'* account of health and disease that some scholars have argued that Plato's name can be associated with a kind of "strong holism" (Stempsey, 2001, p. 204)—an approach to well-being where health is envisioned not merely as *physical* well-being but rather, as "a vision of the good life itself" (op. cit., p. 201). And it is to this holistic conception of health to which I would now like to turn.

3. Caring for the Whole

"This is the mistake some doctors make with their patients.
They try to produce health of body apart from health of soul."
- Plato, *Charmides* 157 b-c

Nowhere is Plato's holistic approach to health made clearer than in the *Charmides*, an early Platonic dialogue devoted to the virtue of moderation (*sophrosyne*), but also, more indirectly, to the subject matters of health and disease. The dialogue begins with an erotically-charged scene where Socrates tries to lure the young Charmides into a conversation about *sophrosyne*. A very attractive and promising young man, Charmides is said to suffer from painful and recurrent headaches. Socrates wants to offer his help to Charmides, but before doing so, Socrates must first fight off a serious case of erection—an erection triggered by Socrates catching a glimpse of Charmides' genitals. Socrates eventually succeeds in regaining his self-control (*sophrosyne*), and informs the young man that he has recently learned a cure for headaches from a Thracian doctor (155d-157a). But Socrates warns Charmides: the remedy he has to propose involves much more than simply applying a substance (a particular leaf) to the head: he who wants to heal must also recite a charm. Without the charm (i.e. the philosophical conversation that is about to take place), the leaf in question will be useless (155e; Brisson, p. 2000). Socrates claims that like all wise doctors, he cannot provide health to anybody without caring for the whole.

> You have probably heard this about good doctors that if you go to them with a pain in the eyes, they are likely to say that they cannot undertake to cure the eyes by themselves, but that it will be necessary to treat the head at the same time if things are also to go well with the eyes (156b-c).

Health problems cannot be addressed solely on the basis of physiological considerations, for such an approach is profoundly limited—a point repeatedly made by critics of Viagra (e.g. Potts, 2008; Loe, 2004).[8] According to Plato, one's particular life circumstances, self-knowledge, socio-economic status, gender, and age must all be taken into consideration when seeking to address someone's health issues. For instance, the importance of one's upbringing, social context *and* biology are all highlighted by Plato in the *Timaeus*, in his account of the causes of 'sexual madness':

> the truth about sexual overindulgence is that it is a disease of the soul caused primarily by the condition of a single stuff which, due to the po-

> rousness of the bones, flows within the body and renders it moist. (…) it is not right to reproach people for [evils done] (…) for no one is willfully evil. A man becomes evil, rather, as a result of one or another corrupt condition of his body *and an uneducated upbringing.* No one who incurs these pernicious conditions would will to have them (*Timaeus* 86d-e; my emphasis).

But if Plato frequently reminds us of the interconnectedness of body and mind, and that of the soul and the city, he definitely *prioritizes* the psychological in his analysis of health and disease. In the *Charmides*, this is underscored when Socrates describes what he has learned from the Thracian doctor: "The soul is the source both of bodily health and bodily disease for the whole man, and these flow from the soul in the same way that their eyes are affected by the head. So it is necessary *first and foremost to cure the soul* if the parts of the head and of the rest of the body are to be healthy" (157b; my italics). We are here presented with the reason that the only patient worth a doctor's time, according to Plato, is he who is ready to change his entire way of life (*7th Letter* 330e): an individual who is ready to engage in a lengthy examination of his soul, and one who is willing to reform it through some patient and regular philosophical exercises (such as the ones the young Charmides is subjected to throughout the dialogue). If some might be tempted to see in this prioritization of the psychological a fair dose of naiveté regarding the concrete physiological or 'mechanical' basis of many illnesses, others might appreciate the timely reminder about how significant a role our cultural, intellectual and socio-political environment might play in creating (and, conversely, in *destroying*) health.

In fact, in the *Charmides* (as in other dialogues), Socrates not only gives precedence to the care of the soul over the care of the body, he seems at times to completely neglect the latter. The leaf (the medication) is never applied to Charmides' head; it never again gets mentioned. Charmides' soul is to be "undressed" but not his body (154e). Indeed, the rest of the dialogue will be concerned entirely with applying 'the charm'—i.e. with treating the headache with the help of the elenchus.

After securing the young man's willful consent (156d), Socrates will subject him to a long dialectical exchange in which Charmides will be forced to realize how little he knows himself, and thus, how ill-equipped he is to govern fellow Athenians. (The choice of Charmides as Socrates' interlocutor in a dialogue about moderation is particularly poignant given the fact that the young man eventually turned into one of the most immoderate tyrants in Athenian history.)[9] As is fairly typical in Plato's early dialogues, the *Charmides* ends in *aporia*, with no satisfying definition of moderation having been found. But the dialogue establishes at least one thing: that true physical well-being calls for much more than the swallowing of a pill or the application of a leaf. Health requires philosophy.

Although many things have been said here about how the wise doctor ought to work his way towards health, we have yet to consider what health is according to Plato. Inspired by Pythagorean and Hippocratic teachings (Carrick, 2001, p. 36–37; Murphy, 2000, p. 294–295; Lidz, 1995, p. 528), Plato conceived of health largely as a matter of proportions and balance between opposing powers—not only between different bodily substances, but also, between internal and external movements, between soul and body. As he writes in the *Timaeus* (87c): "all that is good is beautiful, and what is beautiful is not ill-proportioned. Hence we must take it that if a living thing is to be in good condition, it will be well-proportioned." Now, according to which proportions should health be envisioned? In the *Republic* (e.g. 528a-530a) and *Timaeus* (88d-e), Plato suggests that we ought to take, as our model, the proportions and harmonies that are to be found in the universe and that may be revealed through dialectic and mathematics. (Readers of the *Republic* will recall that it was Plato's hope that these ratios could come to inform not only someone's psychological life, but also, a city's constitution and its music.)

In health (as in all human matters), a mean is best. Indeed, throughout Plato's work, we not only find the idea that excessive sensual indulgence is bad (a claim that will seem reasonable, if unappealing, to baby-boomers), but, more remarkably, the idea that too much physical health is not desirable. Plato insists that disproportionate care for the body and excessive physical health can be important obstacles to the cultivation of virtue (*Republic* 407b-d) and hence, to the good life. This is so not only because an unwarranted amount of time spent on physical training "makes any kind of learning, thought, or private meditation difficult" (407c). The problem is also that excessive concern for the body tends to lead one to worry excessively about one's medical condition. Therefore, one is at risk of imagining some bodily sickness or weakness where none exists, and hence, come to neglect what matters—whether it is leisure, work or philosophy. Given all this, Socrates and the Athenian stranger both insist that the wisest thing to pursue and wish for is a *moderate* amount of physical health:

> The body that deserves to be honored is not the handsome one or the strong or the swift—*nor yet the healthy* (…) and it is certainly not the one with the opposite qualities to all these. (…) *the body which achieves a mean between all these extreme conditions is by far the soundest and best-balanced*, because the one extreme makes the soul bold and boastful, while the other makes it abject and groveling (*Laws* 728d-e; my italics).

Now, lifestyle medicines such as Viagra are marketed in such a way that consumers should come to believe the very opposite. Indeed, "Big Pharma" wants us to be convinced that Plato is simply wrong—that it is absurd to claim that there is a limit to the concern we ought to have for our health, and that it is perfectly rational to seek to prevent the aging process. Indeed, as Barbara Marshall has shown (2002, p. 145), the industry's message could not be clearer: he who refuses the pharmaceutical tools that could allow him to reach 'maximum health' (i.e. the most potent and reliable erections possible, regardless of age or personal circumstances) is either a bad consumer... or plain stupid. To Plato, the inevitable decline in our physical abilities are not be resented or fought against at all costs (financial or otherwise): instead, one ought to welcome old age, for it is in this precious period that one can engage in the best kind of erotic activity: contemplation. (*Republic* 498b-c) If the pharmaceutical industry seeks to convince us that "one cannot rationally choose to decline" physically (Katz & Marshall 2003) and that the most sensible thing to do is to try to stay young forever, this is clearly not the only discourse that is available to us. Plato certainly has something else to propose.

Of course, Plato could not anticipate the intimate connections between an ever-expanding consumerist culture and the resort to lifestyle drugs (although he liked to emphasize a few serious hazards about mixing medicine and money-making).[10] But Plato was certainly able to formulate a claim that seems particularly relevant for us in light of the aggressive promotional campaigns conducted by pharmaceutical and cosmetic manufacturers: that an *excessive* care for the body may come at some cost—in particular, the loss of precious time that could be devoted to more meaningful human pursuits (e.g. *Republic* 407c). My intention here is not to claim that all individuals who resort to cosmetic enhancement or Viagra should pick up philosophy books instead of pills, and that all cases of sexual impotence ought to be disregarded as trivial. Rather, my goal here is only to note that the "Viagra phenomenon" is part of a wider socio-political phenomenon of late capitalism which aims at selling us an ever-increasing amount of sensuous pleasures, material goods and death-defying devices, and that this phenomenon should give us pause. Indeed, as we will now see, more is not always better.

4. 'Less is More': Moderation, Freedom, and Philosophical *Eros*

It would be tempting (if misguided) to gather from all this that Plato associates health with asceticism, virtue with the simple repression of *eros*, and happiness more generally with a sexless life. If this were so, Cephalus would certainly be a healthy and happy man—whereas he is depicted by Plato as the very opposite. What we can gather from the *Republic* is that the old man is struggling with an unbearable fear of death—as his quick exit from the conversation and his comments on the benefits of being wealthy suggest. Indeed, when asked by Socrates what is the "greatest good" he derives from his fortune (made out of selling arms), Cephalus candidly replies that it helps him alleviate his anxiety over death. It can do so because money allows him to purchase the clemency of the gods by repaying the people he has cheated in life. As he puts it:

> You know, Socrates, that when someone thinks his end is near, he becomes frightened and concerned about things he didn't fear before. (...) he is filled with foreboding and fear, and he examines himself to see whether he has been unjust to anyone. If he finds many injustices in his life, he awakes from sleep in terror, as children do, and lives in anticipation of bad things to come (*Republic* 330e-331a).

It does not seem completely unreasonable to gather from such a vivid description and from his own deeds that Cephalus is one of those children, and that he has lived badly his entire life. It is only because "his end is near" that he has started caring about justice (and a limited kind of justice, for that matter). As we saw earlier, Cephalus claims to be a moderate man (*sophron*) and to be at peace with his quiet and pious life—a life that is devoid of excessive drinking and sex. But as his deeds and later words suggest, his moderation is not genuine: his *sophrosyne* is merely accidental. More specifically, it is the result of two things: a terrorizing fear of death, and an inability to maintain an erection (and more generally, an inability to bear any kind of physical exhaustion; 328c). As his comments to Socrates suggest (330e), Cephalus has not lived the life of a truly moderate man—he has cheated, lied, manipulated and abused of many good things. And even at the threshold of death, he seems uninterested in cultivating true *sophrosyne*—which is, as we will see shortly, a kind of *reflective* and *active* self-regulation, rather than the accidental result of events.

It is on that basis that I want to suggest that Cephalus *would* have rushed to his doctor if Viagra had existed in ancient Greece. Contrary to what some scholars have gathered from the *Republic*'s first exchange about justice (e.g. Reeve, 1988; Kakridis, 1948), Cephalus is not *sophron* (and thus cannot be said to be truly sexually moderate either). Cephalus' moderation is not genuine not only because his is unreflective, but also, because it is pursued merely in order to relieve discomfort and suffering (actual or future). In the *Phaedo*, Plato is clear: true *sophrosyne* is not to be pursued in order to increase pleasure, or diminish pain (68e & 82c).

Assuming that Cephalus could manage to find the 'right doctor' (the one we have described in the section above), it is unlikely that he would have been the 'right patient'—i.e. one willing to engage in a meaningful discussion about health, sexual pleasure and their rightful place in the good life. To put it in Foucaultian lingo, Cephalus does not want to know what is a "good use of pleasures": a use of pleasure that is grounded on the agent's careful and informed weighing of several considerations (including those of need and circumstance), and thus, a use that requires much *phronesis* on the part of the individual. Plato would not want Cephalus' sexuality to be ruled by a strict code, one that would explicitly and with 'tyrannical' confidence dictate whether he should once again be allowed to indulge in the pleasures of the flesh (thanks to Viagra) and when, and with what intensity, he should do so. Ideally,

Plato would want Cephalus to regulate for himself his sexual life and to be in control of his body—something which requires reflection. Genuine *sophrosyne* (sexual or otherwise) is not about repressing completely one's passions or about avoiding pleasure, nor is it about achieving some kind of complete purity.[11] Instead, moderation entails the *knowledge* of what is an appropriate amount of sensuous pleasure for one to indulge in, and at what *moment* it is appropriate to do so. More importantly perhaps, moderation also entails the capacity to *resist* the powerful urge to satisfy desires that go beyond that (be they desires for sex, food, money, or power). Put most simply, *sophrosyne* entails self-knowledge and self-control—and it is a virtue that is obtained through one of the noblest battles of all: the battle against oneself (*Laws* 626e). Indeed, contrary to what Callicles claims in the *Gorgias*, *sophrosyne* is not for "the stupid" or for cowards (491e & 492a). And contrary to what Thrasymachus claims in the *Republic*, *sophrosyne* is not the virtue of the impotent: it is not the trait of feeble individuals who are too fearful to ask life for more (344c). Rather, the *sophron* knows that the life of *pleonexia* is an empty sham and that the mastery of self that moderation calls for is the one most indispensable requirement for happiness and for ruling over others (*Gorgias* 494a & 519a; *Alcibiades* 134b-e).

Moderation may require a life-long battle within the self, but it is a battle that brings immense rewards , especially freedom, to the individual. As Foucault puts it in the second volume of his *History of Sexuality*: "sexual moderation is an exercise of liberty, which takes the form of a mastery of the self; this mastery manifests itself in the manner a subject comports himself and restrains himself in the exercise of his virile activity, the way he relates to his self and to others" (Foucault 1984: 125; translation mine). If the moderate man is free, the individual who lacks the capacity to master his appetites and to put his soul in order lives, on the contrary, in utter slavery. Book IX of the *Republic* puts forward that argument, and it does so very graphically: the tyrannical man is presented as one whose sexual longings (the strongest of all desires)[12] get out of control and who, as a result, lives in total wretchedness and fear.

> (…) erotic love lives like a tyrant within him, in complete anarchy and lawlessness as his sole ruler, and drives him, as if he were a city, to dare anything that will provide sustenance for itself and the unruly mob around it (some of whose members have come in from the outside as a result of his keeping bad company, while others have come from within, freed and let loose by his own bad habits) (*Republic* 574e-575a).

Cephalus may leave the room well before Book II of the *Republic* begins, but one could still envision the rest of the work as a long and detailed answer to the old metic's limited worldview and unreflective *sophrosyne*. Indeed, one could suggest that it is not simply with Thrasymachus but also with Cephalus in mind that Plato brings his *Republic* to a close: not only with the very vivid description of the tyrannical, erotic soul of Book IX but also with the myth of Er presented at the very end of the *Republic*.

The myth presents us with the legend of Er, who dies at war but who gets sent back to life to tell human beings about what goes on after death when souls travel to Hades. Er not only recounts the beauties he has witnessed in Hades, but also the horrors: we learn that people whose lives are lived poorly will get reprimanded manifold for each injustice committed on earth (with some never escaping punishment) (615a-c). More importantly for our purposes here, the second part of the myth considers the moment when souls get the opportunity to select their next life. Choices abound: one is free to pick the life of powerful and rich men, playboys, tyrants, animals, athletes, exceptionally virtuous men, plain and unimportant individuals—and the list goes on. Socrates tells Glaucon that

> it is here (…) that a human being faces the greatest danger of all. And because of this, each of us must neglect all other subjects and be most concerned to seek out and learn those that will enable him to distinguish the good life from the bad and always to make the best choice possible in every situation (618c).

We are then told that the first person who gets to choose his next life chooses very poorly: a soul filled with greed decides to select the life of a powerful tyrant. Once he realizes that this life will eventually entail devouring his very own children, the individual curses himself and wails. The crux of the Platonic lesson follows, when we learn from Er that this unhappy individual had lived his previous life *well*: "He was one of those who had come down from heaven, having lived his previous life under an orderly constitution, *where he had participated in virtue through habit and without philosophy*" (619c; my italics). This man's unreflective virtue on earth might have been enough to buy him a temporary voyage through heaven, but it proved insufficient to allow him to make the right choice when faced with his next life.

Now, we will recall that Cephalus is presented to us in the *Republic* as a man whose main reason for acting "justly" (i.e. paying his debts and saying the truth) is his fear of death and fear of punishment. Cephalus does not see why justice (or moderation for that matter) might be good in and of itself—and neither is he interested in figuring out why. Cephalus is no great fan of questions. And thus, like the pitiable soul we are told about in the myth of Er, Cephalus will not fare well in the afterlife. For if Cephalus has any virtue (and it is doubtful that he has any), it is unreflective—or put differently, it is "without philosophy" (*Republic* 619c).

What this means is that, were he given a prescription for Viagra, Cephalus could hardly benefit from it according to Plato: he would in all likelihood abuse of the little blue pills and hence subject his aged body (and perhaps his wife and courtesans?) to poor treatment. More significantly, Cephalus would be harmed by Viagra because the possibility to engage once more in feasts and orgies would take him further away from the contemplative life. For Plato, only philosophy could (potentially) relieve Cephalus of his true diseases: his fear of death and his poor way of living. If the encounter between the old metic and Socrates is Cephalus' "last chance" to live well the last years of his life, it is, more importantly, Cephalus' "last chance" to engage in what will be necessary to make the right decision concerning his *next* life. No medicine or technology can help the old metic figure out what is "the most important thing, namely, the good life and the bad one" (*Republic* 578c).

Given the great likelihood that Cephalus would abuse of Viagra (in light of his lack of moderation), would it not be more sensible simply to ban the blue pill in the ideal city, the *kallipolis*? To put it differently: faced with the reality of Viagra, would it not have been Plato's spontaneous response to forbid the blue pill and thus to forcefully compel the old man to run after truth rather than after reliable erections? There are many good grounds to believe that the answer should be no. For one thing, a mere ban would do little to encourage Cephalus to pursue philosophy and work on his character; it would merely prevent (potential) harm, not necessarily do any good. As we are frequently reminded in various Platonic dialogues, law and coercion are ultimately insufficient for instilling moderation and health in citizens.[13] Persuasion and education are, for Plato, the most significant and desirable ways to lead souls to the good life—not compulsion. After all, "nothing taught by force stays in the soul" (*Republic* 536e). Besides, beyond Cephalus, Plato would probably have agreed that some individuals who are in possession of a fair degree of moderation could *benefit* from the pill, under the right circumstances. The 'benefits' Plato would care most about are not those tied to the enhanced sensuous pleasures provided by the pill, nor those tied to one's self-esteem and marital happiness (an issue to which we will return in the conclusion). Rather, Plato would welcome Viagra in light of the opportunity provided by the pill to reinforce one's virtue by choosing to swallow up Viagra (or not) at the appropriate time and for the right reasons. Put differently, Viagra could serve as a 'test' for one's virtue—a role similar to that attributed to wine at the beginning of the *Laws* (649d-650b).

The life of the *sophron* will no doubt sound excessively 'monkish' to many contemporary ears. Foucault is far from alone in having identified in Platonic moderation a kind of *ethos* that has significant ascetic overtones.[14] Nevertheless, I am not convinced that it is entirely appropriate to suggest, as Peter Steinberger has, that what Socrates has to propose to Cephalus is a "*thorough* and principled asceticism" (Steinberger 1995: 191; my italics). While there is no doubt that Socrates seeks to convince his interlocutors—young or old, potent or not—that an unreflective hedonism is the best recipe for injustice and unhappiness, Socrates remains a deeply erotic man. And by this I do not simply want to suggest that Socrates is driven by a strong erotic longing for wisdom—a reasonable claim made by most Plato scholars and one Peter

Steinberger would have no qualms with. More controversially perhaps, I also want to suggest that sexual/bodily longings are a significant part of Socrates' being, and that these longings are not wholly disconnected from his philosophic pursuit. Put differently, contemplation is an erotic activity in a very bodily and concrete way according to Plato. In my view, we ought to regard as significant the fact that Socrates is portrayed in the Platonic dialogues as an individual who is physically attracted to those he is keenest on enlightening (e.g. Charmides and Alcibiades) and that his young interlocutors are often similarly stirred. One might object that Socrates never actually satisfies his sexual or sensuous cravings: he is presented to us (most vividly in the *Symposium*)[15] as the arch-model of *sophrosyne*—an impossible model to emulate. Nevertheless, even if Socrates' love of beautiful bodies is made subservient to the demands of soul-craft, his *eros* remains a spur to it. True Platonic Viagra may be addressed to the soul, but bodily yearnings and pleasures are not completely disregarded—kisses and caresses are, rather, to be channeled towards "what is fine and beautiful" (*Republic* 403b).[16]

5. The Limits of Platonic Thought

But is it not "too late" for Cephalus to engage in anything akin to philosophy, as Pierre Javet has suggested? (Javet 1982: 244) When death is so near, when one's physical capacities have so drastically declined, and when one's entire existence has been so utterly unreflective, it would seem that the most sensible thing to do would be to make what remains of life as *pleasant* as possible. On the basis of such logic, one could suggest that what Cephalus should do is to gulp down a few blue pills, disregard the admonitions of his guest regarding health and the good life, and simply go on trying to acquire psychological tranquility by performing religious sacrifices. But this conclusion would betray many important Platonic insights: that old age can be the most fruitful time to pursue contemplation; that the only true sin is ignorance; that health cannot be achieved without caring for one's soul; and that any reflective pursuit is better than none.

But while it may never be undesirable or "too late" to care for one's soul (and thus to work one's way to better health), the task at hand seems enormous if not unfeasible. Indeed, the demands put on the shoulders of the good Platonic 'patient' (like those put on the shoulders of the good doctor) are extraordinary. One must not only live according to a strict discipline and shun all political and monetary ambitions; one must also be willing to take full responsibility for one's health and one's entire way of life (*Republic* 426a). Our individual responsibility entails daily exertion at self-cultivation, and it also entails the moral duty to seek treatment for oneself when appropriate. Indeed, in the *Republic*, we learn that it is not up to doctors (of the soul and of the body) to go to the homes of the sick, but rather, the very opposite: "The natural thing is for the sick person, rich or poor, to knock at the doctor's door, and for anyone who needs to be ruled to knock at the door of the one who can rule him" (*Republic* 489c).

Towards those who shun their responsibilities and opt to indulge in a life of complete injustice, licentiousness or idleness, Plato is absolutely unforgiving: "Medicine isn't intended for such people and they shouldn't be treated, not even if they're richer than Midas" (408b). The cold logic presented by Plato in these passages of the *Republic* is unsettling (and it is even more so when Plato applies it to people *born* with physical disabilities). It also seems to be quite reminiscent of a type of reactionary discourse offered by neo-conservatives—particularly when the latter present us with their viewpoints on health care costs, morality, and personal responsibility. But there is one significant difference between Platonic thought and contemporary reactionary discourse: Plato makes his harsh pronouncements about individual responsibility towards health within works in which he dreams of cities where poverty would have no place and where the greatest responsibility of legislators would not be the maximization of a nation's GDP or the reduction of a state's public spending, but rather, the provision of the best education possible. Plato's perspective on health matters might be said to suffer from a serious lack of compassion, but it is not naïve: Plato knows that poverty, education and various socio-economic factors have a tremendous impact on people's physical and psychological well-being. If it is true that Plato would not have had enthusiasm for lifestyle drugs (for the reasons discussed above), I have suggested in this essay that he would probably not have banned them. Rather, he would have insisted that an ideal city should work its way towards better health not from 'without' (with laws and bans) but 'from within'—through education and patient, rational persuasion. Indeed, this essay has suggested that while Socrates would not have stopped Cephalus from resorting to Viagra, he would nevertheless have tried—with the help of a charm, with the help of words—to convince him to do otherwise.

Socrates' advice to Cephalus would have been informed by two considerations: first, the fact that the old metic did not possess genuine moderation; second, the fact that the blue pill would have done nothing for Cephalus' real sickness—his anxiety over death. One consideration that would never have crossed Socrates' mind, however, is the welfare of Cephalus' wife and the happiness of their marriage. If we know very little about Cephalus—apart from the fact that he was a foreigner, that he was rich, and that he had democratic sympathies—we know even less about his wife. (Nails, 2002; Steinberger, 1996) We do not know, for instance, whether she was still alive when Socrates had his conversation with the old Cephalus. But even if she had been around and healthy when Plato wrote the *Republic* some time around 390 B.C., it is very unlikely that her name would have figured in the dialogue, and this silence would not be due to misogyny. The greatest philosophical problems—justice and the good life—are never approached by Plato via considerations of an individual's happiness. In his view, the city's good is the only thing that truly matters: civic harmony and relations are paramount, and private attachments are worthy at best of mistrust and at worst, of scorn and fear.

It is here that we meet one of the gravest limitations of Plato's conception of well-being and love (*eros*): his disregard for the worth and significance of private, particular relationships.[17] Socrates *should* have asked Cephalus about his wife; he *should* have—at least briefly—considered the impact of Cephalus' impotence on their marital relationship. But such considerations are simply not part of the Platonic imaginary (it is probably safe to say that they are not part of the Greek imaginary more generally). Of course, if asked by Socrates for her own thoughts on old age and sexuality, Cephalus' wife may not necessarily have expressed sorrow over the death of the couple's sex life. She may have voiced her gratitude for the "freedom" and tranquility brought about by the erectile difficulties of her husband; or she may have cheered at her *own* departed libido—a view that peppered American news media recently when the U.S. Food and Drug Administration released its report about the questionable safety of Boehringer Ingelheim's 'pink' Viagra. In language reminiscent of the old Cephalus, one female *New York Times* reader observed: "One of the greatest benefits of the postmenopausal life has been the diminution of slavery to sexual desire. I have felt so much freer and lighter (...) [I] cannot image wanting to reignite all that yearning, depression and frustration again."[18] *Plus ça change...*

Notes

1. All Plato citations (including those from the *7th Letter*) are taken from the following translation: Plato, *Complete Works*, John M. Cooper & D.S. Hutchinson ed. (Indianapolis: Hackett, 1997).
2. Indeed, it is said here by Cephalus that the *majority* of old men resent their sexual impotence. One could also see Cicero's *On Old Age* (1923) for comments on the resentment caused by impotence, and Hippocrates (1984) for brief discussions of impotence and more importantly, for proposed *remedies*. For the imprecise claim that impotence used to be accepted with grace, see for instance Katz & Marshall 2003, or Marshall 2006: 346.
3. But compare with page 29, where Rosen refers to Cephalus as a "moderate hedonist."
4. In the *Republic* (444e), virtue is also defined as "a kind of health," and in his *7th Letter*, Plato draws close analogies between the physician and the statesman (e.g. 330e-331d). For a detailed discussion of medicine and health as *metaphors* in Plato, see Lidz (1995) and Ménissier (1995).
5. Contrary to some scholars, I take Plato's feminism seriously; there is no good reason why Plato's ideal city and second-best city could not have included female doctors. See the *Republic's* Book V and the *Laws* 781a, 805a-d, 814a-c for some of Plato's most important statements regarding gender equality.
6. The *Laws* is perhaps the exception here: homosexuality is disparaged; sexuality is circumscribed; the sex life of athletes is put under much scrutiny, etc. But even

in that work, Plato insists that, ideally, laws and fear should not be the *primary* motives constraining and informing sexual practices but rather, that education should.

7. Callicles' position is most explicitly stated at *Gorgias* 491e-492a: "the man who'll live correctly ought to allow his own appetites to get as large as possible and not restrain them. And when they are as large as possible he ought to be competent to devote himself to them by virtue of his bravery and intelligence, and to fill them with whatever he may have an appetite for at the time." For the most emblematic Thrasymachean statement, see *Republic* 343c-344c.
8. See also *Timaeus* 88a-e & *Phaedrus* 270b.
9. The other interlocutor of Socrates (i.e. Critias) will also be a major player in the Thirty Tyrants' regime. For details about these individuals, see Nails 2002.
10. See the most revealing passage at *Republic* 342d.
11. Only in the *Phaedo* does Plato put forward an understanding of *sophrosyne* that has great ascetic overtones. E.g. 82c-83c.
12. E.g. *Republic* 403a
13. E.g. *Laws* 835e; *7th Letter* 330d. But compare with *Laws* 783a.
14. Foucault (1984) sees in the late Plato the contours of a (proto-Christian) ideal of abstinence and sensuous tranquility. See for instance pages 314 and 316.
15. The most explicit passages are to be found at 219c-220d.
16. Sexual encounters (those that are geared entirely towards pleasure) are not forbidden in Plato's utopian city, the *kallipolis*. For one explicit passage, see 461c.
17. On the issue of marital friendship and reciprocity, see the chapter of Kevin Guilfoy in this volume.
18. *New York Times* online (June 17, 2010). www.nytimes.com/2010/06/17/business/17sexpill.html (accessed June 17, 2010).

Two

DIOGENES OF SINOPE GETS HARD ON VIAGRA

Robert Vuckovich

1. Introduction

There is an occasion when Diogenes of Sinope encounters a man who has an obvious erectile dilemma. Given the details, it may be best to call it a deficiency as opposed to a dysfunction. As the story goes: "A eunuch of bad character had inscribed on his door the words, 'Let nothing evil enter.' 'How then', [Diogenes] asked, 'is the master of the house to get in?'" (Diogenes Laertius, 1991, p. 41) Even though it is speculative to determine whether this individual's character contributed to his being castrated, or whether the castration resulted from something either punitive or accidental, one notices that this man has a problem. Diogenes' question points to the eunuch's inability to recognize how the restriction that he establishes applies to him as well as other evildoers. At issue here is the impotence of the eunuch's moral reasoning. Yet with that same question, Diogenes draws attention to the eunuch's inability to participate in penetrative sex.

The reference to how the eunuch is to "get in" relates sylleptically to his inability to perform most penetrative activities. Castration not only creates a physiological deficiency, it too takes much of a man's sexual potency away. Impotence of this extreme nature is the death of a man and his sex drive. Poking fun at this predicament, Diogenes demonstrates that the eunuch has nothing to offer. Further injury is added to the psychological state of the eunuch when Diogenes addresses him as "the master," for his ability to partake in penetrative intercourse is way beyond his control.

It is highly doubtful that the eunuch's form of impotence could ever benefit from any pharmaceutical treatment. Restoration of the eunuch's erection would most definitely involve a transplant and subsequent medical treatments to establish real sensations in a surrogate penis. No wonder drug would ever be available to help a eunuch naturally grow a new appendage. And Viagra clearly is no such drug. So then, would Diogenes say anything less critical or humorous to those using Viagra for erectile dysfunction issues whom have naturally become inoperative?

2. Indecent Behavior, Prescriptive Promises, and Penetrating Concerns

Unfortunately, well over two thousand years separate the philosopher from Viagra's inception. Any sort of response from Diogenes would have to be based on his views on human sexual relations. There are plenty of accounts and anecdotes about his ideas that can provide an adequate viewpoint of how other persons should conduct their personal lives and deal with sexual matters. For instance, since no sympathy is given to the eunuch for being unable to "get in," it seems unlikely that Diogenes would voice any concern for those just wanting to get it up in order to get it on. Some people might think to the contrary, that he would be supportive of matters pertaining to erectile dysfunction, because this character, an ancient version of Dr. Giles Brindley,[1] gained a reputation for being quite handy with his penis. Public masturbation stands out as one of Diogenes' most notable exploits (D. L., 1991, pp. 47, 71). This level of concentration on and manipulation of the penis should indicate that he has no reservations about keeping it active regardless of time and place. It is as though sexual gratification through penile stimulation is of the utmost importance for a guy. Philosophically, though, this conventionally lewd act constitutes an example of self-sufficiency (*autarkeia*).

Understanding this seemingly self-absorbed approach to what Diogenes deems as a natural form of human sexual expression requires one to avoid seeing the masturbatory episode as a case of uncontrollable wantonness. Consider that during this exploit, his expressed wish relates to the difficulty of sating his hunger by a similar means, for he prefers not to depend too much on external resources. *Autarkeia*, incidentally, does not apply to every human appetite, making an individual somewhat dependent on certain activities. The ease with which sexual gratification is achieved reveals something more about Diogenes' perspective on sexual relations as a whole in that the urgency to sate his sexual appetite may not always be in conjunction with a desire for sexual pleasure.

Dispelling pleasure seems counterintuitive to why a man would devote time and effort to stroking his penis. The Roman physician, Galen, observes that Diogenes exhibits a disciplined effort to expel pleasure while masturbating.[2] Medically speaking, "he indulged in sexual relations, since he wanted to get rid of the inconvenience caused by the retention of sperm, (…) not for the pleasure associated with this elimination" (Galen, 1976, p.184). This masturbatory act functions as a substitute for an intended intimate encounter with a woman, one specifically arranged to provide sexual favors, and denies him any mutually physical gratification. "My hand," Diogenes claims, "was faster than you in celebrating the bridal night" (Galen, 1976, p. 185). This insulting comment to a courtesan not only means that he can manage on his own, but that he can disregard the celebratory time of penetrative intercourse despite having recently had a desire for it. Curbing this passion as such signifies discipline. *Autarkeia* is not an automatic reaction to fulfilling an individual person's desire, because when Diogenes put his mind to it, masturbation operates as an exercise (*askēsis*) in managing his sexual urges. Exercising this type of self-control allows him to keep his mind content and his sex organ operational without overdoing it solitarily or licentiously with others.

In this capacity, Diogenes does not appear to be a likely spokesman for Viagra. He apparently has no erectile dysfunction (ED), especially when he is able to perform as he sees fit. It is doubtful then that Diogenes' method would be essential for staving off impotence. Yet a point worth noting from that episode is that the mental component behind a man's sexual performance determines whether he is impotent. "The problem in most cases of impotence is not in the man's penis, but in his brain, in his perception of his sexuality (…) impotence is most often due to anxiety and to the fear of failure to perform sexually (…)" (Llewellyn-Jones, 1987, p. 193). Never experiencing any real distress relating to his public one-man sex show, Diogenes is quite mindful of his sexual nature. But also arising out of that particular episode is a more developed perspective on how the sexual nature of others should operate. A. A. Long notices how "[Diogenes'] own behavior [serves] as a way of commenting on human nature's possibilities and limitations" (Long, 1996, p. 33; modifications mine). Instead of functioning like a medical practician, Diogenes would likely prescribe his own philosophical take on human sexuality and its moral dilemmas in relation to how Viagra influences more than just a man's penis.

Only in the case of the eunuch does one see Diogenes show no genuine concern for a man unable to perform sexually. Again, Viagra could never restore a eunuch's sex drive because of his incapacity of having an erection. But the drug is capable of forming a sizable change in a man's life. Facilitating blood flow to a limp penis is physiologically all that Viagra does. So upon the medicinal success of taking one pill, an impotent man typically regains the use of his sexual instrument and can then participate in any sort of penetrative intercourse when he desires. A revitalized penis becomes a psychological boost for the man, because, according to Potts et al., Viagra "also [enhances] his self-image, his lifestyle and his relationships with others in more personal ways" (Potts et al., 2003, p. 698, 699; modification mine). These additional perks may make someone impotent even more tempted to try the drug. It is difficult to be skeptical about such enhancements when current scientific research finds "high satisfaction" among a majority of those relying on "the treatment" (Chevret-Méasson et al., 2009, p. 766). So should there be any concern about using a drug that enhances sexual performance?

Given positive findings associated with Viagra treatment, it would seem fair for Diogenes to challenge the pharmaceutical approach to dealing with impotence. Diogenes never calls into question the use of ancient remedies or medical practices. Yet he does get angry at health conscious men who hypocritically consume that which is "the detriment of health" (D. L., 1991, p. 31). Men's appetites take hold of their better judgment, interfering with the prospect of healthy living. So Diogenes has no reason to direct blame squarely on what is consumed. Viagra is not a mind numbing substance like a narcotic. Or, is it? The promise of enhancements after taking the drug is quite alluring. If Viagra treatment does fulfill the expectations of its users, impotent men will depend on it for continued sexual gratification. And when it comes time to deal with ED, the male mindset is, as Derek Llewellyn-Jones reminds, already in a distressed state. The issue existentially becomes one where an individual can consider whether the lifestyle change a pill may offer is actually fulfilling.

Even before a man can benefit from Viagra, he needs to consult with a physician. At this preliminary stage of treatment, a physician may pose a problem for the patient, for there are consequences to prescribing a life altering medication. Eugene V. Boisaubin and Lawrence B. McCullough point to how the relation between a physician and one's patient determines whether the concerns about impotency are appropriately addressed. Proper treatment of ED begins when the physician gains "more knowledge about the patient's sexual behavior and its impact upon the partner(s)" (Boisaubin et al., 2004, p. 742). This honest, sensitive disclosure reveals how ethically responsible a physician has to be when treating ED and thinking about the patient's sexual expectations. The patient's best interest is what matters most.

Not having any consideration for their patients troubles Diogenes about physicians. In a specific anecdote focusing on the abuse of authority, abuse that is also sexual in nature, Diogenes cautions a naïve patient from being mistreated. "When Didymon, who was a rake, was once treating a girl's eye, 'Beware', says Diogenes, 'lest the oculist instead of curing the eye should ruin the pupil'" (D. L., 1991, p. 71). It is apparent that the girl's medical condition is completely unrelated to what a man with ED experiences, and the so-called physician, Didymon, has a disposition uncharacteristic of the physicians whom Boisaubin and McCullough have in mind, but the point about receiving improper medical care is a violation of the patient. Indeed, the sexual violation of the girl is something Diogenes finds disturbing, but what also upsets him is the misleading sense of trust that develops between the authoritative physician and the compliant patient, which inadvertently conflicts with the notion that the patient is supposed to benefit from medical attention or the physician's guidance. Note the sylleptical style in which Diogenes talks about how "the pupil" will be ruined, simply because she is ignorant of the oculist's true interest. This specific incident represents a serious injustice whereby a patient unwittingly depends on an unsupportive physician.

Examining once again the prescriptive concerns Boisaubin and McCullough have about Viagra, one has to realize that, similar to Diogenes' oculist, undesirable sexual relations happen among Viagra users. As mentioned earlier, a physician must be made aware of a "patient's sexual behavior" in order for the treatment of ED have any success. The reasoning behind this concern relates to the enhanced lifestyle an erect penis gives. Put otherwise, once a man has a functional erection, that penis will assuredly partake in penetrative activities. Penetration and erection go hand in hand when it comes to Viagra use. There is the fear that in the pursuit of sexual satisfaction, some Viagra users will engage "in [behaviors] that are reliably predicted to be dangerous to others" (Boisaubin et al., 2004, p. 744; modification mine; see also Del Casino Jr., 2007, p. 909).

Sexually transmitted diseases (STDs) first come to mind when danger is mentioned, but contracting them tends to be an issue when the Viagra user either has previously contracted an STD and resumes having unprotected penetrative intercourse with a partner(s) without revealing his condition or has intercourse with a partner who fails to disclose that he, or she, is infected. The ethical dilemma in these circumstances has less to do with Viagra use than the individual responsibilities of having unprotected sex when at least one person is infected and does not inform the partner. Toning down their concern about these dangers, Boisaubin and McCullough do not believe that Viagra sets off such careless behaviors. Instead, "some (…) consequences [arising from the interest to have penetrative intercourse after the man takes Viagra] may be unwelcome" (Boisaubin et al., 2004, p. 744; addition mine).

Going back to Diogenes' encounter with the oculist, one realizes that sexual deviancy may be a part of the renewed sexual relations of some Viagra users. With a penis restored back to life, as it were, a man's desire to have penetrative intercourse tends to adopt a domineering attitude. Consider that Didymon, by Diogenes' estimation, is most interested in seducing the girl as opposed to "curing the eye." Accordingly, their relation lacks any mutual foundation, in that the girl depends on Didymon to cure her eye, while the oculist focuses on the girl to tweak his interest. She should not be obliged to serve his bodily needs in exchange for his professional service. Similarly, some Viagra users in an attempt to re-establish sexual relations with a partner, or partners, disregard the "important biopsychological interests of [their] sexual partners [who may be] at risk in unpredictable and perhaps harmful ways, for example vaginal injury or increased stress from unwanted sexual overture" (Boisaubin et al., 2004, p. 744; modifications mine). Many female partners of Viagra users in one study have voiced their concern about performing unwanted favors routinely (Potts et al., 2003. pp. 709, 711). So what Diogenes' oculist has in common with some Viagra users is the overwhelming desire to have penetrative intercourse while disregarding their partners' sexual interests, let alone their well-being. The convenience of getting an instant hard-on with Viagra seems closely tied to the idea that a man using Viagra has not only the ability to fulfill his sexual appetite, but to do as he pleases.

3. Sexual Passion, Sexual Freedom, and Sexual Discipline

Everything said about Diogenes up till now seems to present him in both a respectable and crass manner. As indicated earlier, he values *autarkeia*, because it constitutes an expression of individual accomplishment as well as freedom. The liberty to masturbate when a man's urge strikes should then be proof that Diogenes fully supports the freedom of physical expression. Incidentally, he deems "Freedom of speech" to be "the most beautiful thing" (D. L., 1991, p. 71). Just like the difference that Diogenes notices between the appetite for sex and hunger while masturbating, freedoms pertaining to one's body may not be as beautiful as its oratory counterpart. Examining Diogenes' attachment to personal freedom, John Rist suggests that bodily urges for sexual relations tend to be undesirable. Philosophers with Diogenes' disposition, Rist claims, realize "that the basic human urge to sexuality provides an opportunity for such free relationships. Naturally, [Diogenes would] master (...) this urge, as of all others" (Rist, 1969, p. 61; modifications mine). Once again, one sees how the practice of individual discipline (*askēsis*) aims to tame sexual urges. Otherwise, giving in to them would distort such "free relationships," emphasizing a form of ethical egoism, whereby a "man naturally acts for self-interest, and (...) since he cannot do otherwise, (...) he [goes] with the flow and not (...) oppose it" (Yoos, 1985, p. 58; modification mine). It is at this juncture a sizeable mistake to think that Diogenes' antics and perspectives, however provocative and suggestive, promote selfishness and licentiousness.

The preservation of "free relationships" amounts to restricting the opportunities an individual has in exploiting them. Although it might seem odd for Diogenes to want to restrict personal freedom, there is good reason for doing so. Liberties that lead to carefree behavior can be disruptive to both a person's physical and mental state. Physiologically, too much blood is required to nourish an erect penis, perhaps causing the brain to go hungry during long periods of arousal and penetrative intercourse. However, this phenomenon occurs when a man either is naturally excited or pumped up on Viagra. Avoiding such a state becomes a personal exercise of one's freedom. According to Luis E. Navia, when *askēsis* establishes stability in a person, it enables one to "cleanse the mind of confusion and obfuscation, and the body of detrimental substances and unnatural habits, and succeed in strengthening the will" (Navia, 2005, p. 148). The unabashed freedom to pursue sexual relations, viz., lust, is a human urge that verges on being unnatural, because it renders the male mind impotent due to its excessive concentration on sexual pleasure. For Diogenes, "bad men obey their lusts as servants obey their masters" (D. L., 1991, p. 69). Being a master in such an instance consists of not being influenced by one's passions. Lust, as in the case of Didymon, directs a man's interest to another person and forms a dependency where the targeted person becomes compliant so as to stimulate and gratify the penis. The human body receives far too much attention when one's passion for sex assumes so much control. Not letting his sexual appetite get the better of him, Diogenes puts his mind into action by thinking of his stomach while masturbating. Vital to him is the individual need to train in tandem one's mind and body, for they "secure freedom of movement for virtuous deeds" (D. L., 1991, p. 71). Greater individual freedom flourishes when one frees oneself from the habit of satisfying one's appetite at the expense of another person, which may in turn help establish relationships that are much freer and virtuous in nature.

Sexual intercourse is not completely frowned upon by either the partners' of Viagra users or Diogenes. Yet, as mentioned earlier, several women found penetrative intercourse at times too much to take. With the introduction of Viagra into their lives, women's "sexual [relationships…] involved an increased frequency and/or prolonged durations of sexual relations, and/or repeated penile-vaginal sex over several hours (…)" (Potts et al., 2003, p. 703; modification mine). Viagra in those cases has influenced men to become more determined to partake in penetrative intercourse and made women more accommodating. Certain ads for the drug even market this polar dualism (Simon-Maeda, 2008, p. 32). Placing such demands on a partner puts a strain on the relationship and makes coitus both desired from one vantage point and despised from another, all because the penis is fuelled and ready for action. It is as though this reactivated member creates some psychological friction between men and women's interest in sexual relations. The drug has an influential part in that division, because without it, penile penetration is not possible or, some may think, pleasurable. One observation of this problem claims that "the importance placed on Viagra for men [is] another instance of men's sexual desires and pleasures being prioritized over women's" (Potts et al., 2003, p. 713; modification mine). As Viagra nourishes the penis with new life, it is seen as the agent, or a third party, needed to initiate intimacy, bringing a man and a woman together. Yet it also stands in the way. Similar to how lust forms one-sided, though desired, sexual relations in the minds of men, the pharmaceutical involvement tips the scales in the men's favor by emphasizing their need for penetrative intercourse. Opposing this unfairness, Diogenes treats both sexual interests on mutual terms by downplaying the male's interest and liberating the female's.

Having acted as a meddlesome third party in Didymon's lustful attempt to prod a young female, Diogenes puts his own passions to the test when faced with an identical situation. Sexual and moral tensions build up in Diogenes when he encounters a seemingly open invitation to indulge sexually. As Diogenes Laertius reports, "he saw a woman kneeling before the gods in an ungraceful attitude, and wishing to free her of superstition (…) he came forward and said, 'Are you not afraid, my good woman, that a god may be standing behind you?—for all things are full of his presence—and you may be put to shame?'" (D. L., 1991, p. 39) Not only does Diogenes' question admonish the woman for appearing promiscuous, it simultaneously cautions her about how she may be perceived as a receptacle for an assertive man who longs to take full advantage of her gracelessness. Her liberation manifests itself when she is made aware of how she can, recognizing herself as a "good woman," avoid sexual exploitation by not catering to another's appetite. Potts et al. would welcome Diogenes non-sexual intrusion, for "many [present day] women [experience] some pressure to 'make the most of a tablet', if not for their own pleasure (...)" (Potts et al., 2003, p. 705; modifications mine). The reference to superstition becomes Diogenes' manner of debunking the genuflectory attitude that a woman may adopt in her sexual relations with men. Without examining this anecdote to any great length, Marie-Odile Goulet-Cazé dismisses any religious practice or belief connected to what Diogenes is advocating here (Goulet-Cazé, 1996, p. 73). It is in Diogenes' estimation a case where no good man would stick his, using Potts et al.'s words, "sexual desires and pleasures" to a woman unannounced and without consent.

Another way of ensuring that this woman's liberation is made successful occurs when a man, as Diogenes does, frees himself from wanting to disgrace her. Diogenes takes the initiative to confront the kneeling woman about her position in life and nothing more. Most of his question refers to the divine stature exhibited by a man. His manner of thinking suggests that since the kneeling woman has positioned herself ungracefully, or provocatively, a man will most likely get aroused by viewing such a display. Diogenes is no exception, for his reference to "all things are full of his presence" seems to refer to his getting a hard on, which signifies a natural attraction to what he sees and a readiness for penetrative intercourse. But he dissociates himself from this tempting situation. Not all gods care to stoop so low, as it were. *Askēsis*, an exercise in personal restraint, enables Diogenes to suppress his immediate sexual interest in penetrating the kneeling woman from behind. There tends to be a concern about the woman's readiness for penetrative intercourse, for in a frequently discussed anecdote about a "community of wives," Diogenes favors that a woman gives her "consent" to be in a relation she may be pressured to participate in (D. L., 1991, p. 75).[3] This show of respect for personal choice is unlike the treatment most of the women of the Potts et al.'s study group experienced with medicinally enhanced horny men.

Relating this episode of Diogenes' self-control to how some Viagra users engage their partners sexually does beg the question as to whether he would be more critical of their behavior as opposed to the drug itself. The episode with the kneeling woman represents his scorn towards sexual encounters that are both casual and exploitive. So does Viagra use contribute to similar encounters? Andrea Simon-Maeda spots "Viagra's usefulness for recreational sex" in a 2004 advertisement, which depicts a man's taking delight in doing things his own way (Simon-Maeda, 2008, p. 34). Demonizing the Viagra user in this manner has as much to do with inflating his pride as it does with stiffening his penis. Pharmaceutical advancements often are socially and morally inadequate in dealing with the unpredictable consequences of patients' activities, for according to a study about Viagra use and marketing in Japan, "Viagra and recreational sex are not a topic of 'scientific' scrutiny" (Castro-Vázquez, 2006, p. 125). Viagra's involvement with recreational sex has detached it from the initial pharmaceutical approach to treating impotence.

Dysfunction is now replaced by a combination of dissatisfaction and exploration. A man can abandon the same old partner in order to cultivate unexplored fancies. According to a report in the *British Medical Bulletin* about the company that manufactures the drug, "Pfizer [has] entered into the recreational lifestyle scene promoting Viagra for younger men who like to party [which] may encourage the increase of high-risk sexual behavior" (Rubin et al., 2009, p. 59; modifications mine; see also Marshall and Katz, 2002, p. 61). Boisaubin and McCullough's earlier concern about dangerous sexual practices may not be worth ignoring after all. While some academes, like Rist (1969, p. 60) and Timothy Madigan, are of the view that Diogenes advocates the "enjoyment of worldly pleasures (including sexual activities of all sorts)" (Madigan, 2008, p. 16), one must take note that the younger generation are better off with a more self-gratifying venture than taking unnecessary risks. "One day observing a youth studying philosophy, [Diogenes] said, 'Well done, Philosophy, that thou divertest admirers of bodily charms to the real beauty of the soul'" (D. L., 1991, p. 61; modification mine). Too much emphasis on the body or other bodies once again leads to the unhealthy development of an individual. Receiving Diogenes' approbation--a rare phenomenon, the student's mental exercise gets him to concentrate and appreciate that which has no affinity to superficial physical gratifications. The youth is taking time to work his mind. Diogenes' criticism of lust's taking control of men's rational faculties can be directed at Viagra, because the drug, in a rhetorical rethinking of the 2004 ad, is directly behind such devilish recreations. There is no need for moral reflection once a man has taken the drug and then has penetrative intercourse regardless of whom his partner is. It is time for a revitalized man to put his penis into action and rejoice. Besides, it is so doubtful that Pfizer would ever profit from promoting philosophy as it does with Viagra.

4. Active Libido and Old Age

Older men, if our attention can be directed to the other end of the age spectrum, remain the primary target clientele for Viagra, for their need of support is paramount and their interest in sex is typically intact. Since many parts of the male body begin to function below their peak performance as time goes on, Viagra acts as the proverbial crutch for the less rigid and ED afflicted penis. The pill does even more, in that it enables an old man to remain naturally human. There tends to be the misguided "idea [that] old people caressing, copulating, and enjoying their sexuality is considered obscene and repugnant" (Llewellyn-Jones, 1987, p. 276; modification mine). Viagra use can be seen as establishing social acceptance among those who have difficulties in seeing the aged as having appetites and participating in sexual activities. So would the aged be hounded by Diogenes and subjected to his crass commentary about their intimate exploits? A sympathetic side to the ancient critic emerges when one looks at his perspective on aging and the aged.

Not having the freedom to do as one has grown accustomed to bothers Diogenes somewhat. When asked about what he regards as "wretched in life," his response is: "An old man destitute" (D. L., 1991, p. 53). *Autarkeia*, as might be surmised, becomes noticeably difficult for the aged. Relying on assistance of some form becomes commonplace. Even Diogenes relies on a cane when the infirmities of his later years take hold (D. L., 1991, p. 25). But what does he have to say about old men and their appetites, if any, for sex? Nothing descriptive about the sexual activities of older men stands out, unless a re-examination of the incident involving Didymon's attempted seduction of a young girl is in order. Additionally, Diogenes does not elaborate on the conditions that make an old man destitute. It is not as though impotence or the lack of penetrative intercourse is a topic of interest for the aged in Diogenes' time. Consider on a related note that the opening discussion in Plato's *Republic* touches on how old age brings about relief from human passions. Sharing the sentiment on sexual relations expressed by the aging poet, Sophocles, Socrates' first interlocutor, Cephalus, has discovered that "old age brings peace and freedom from all such things. When the appetites relax and cease to importune us, (…) we escape from many mad masters" (Plato, 1992, p. 4). Old age disables a man's urge to pursue sex. Yet this disability brings about a freedom from "bodily charms" and physical relations and delights. Although Cephalus does possess the financial means to support himself for the duration of his life, is Diogenes so inclined to call Cephalus destitute given what the latter has said about escaping the control of his sexual appetites? Cephalus is quite content with losing the appetites responsible for his losing control. Thought out differently, he has become psychologically impotent, or rather, defiant of his sexual passions, not physiologically impotent. There is no need then to factor in Diogenes' rebuke of Didymon when examining Cephalus, because the old man's libido no longer takes hold of him as it did early in his life. Missing out on sexual relations would not on this account make an old man destitute or make his life wretched.

Viagra could not be in the market if men with Sophocles' and Cephalus' mindset to passively brush off their desires without concern were the norm. It is fair to question whether their attitudes about getting old and losing interest in sex are natural. Perhaps they are odd exceptions. Several modern day studies acknowledge that "sexual interest [remains] moderate to high for the majority of women and men" (Hillman, 2008, p. 290; modification mine). Not all "mad masters" are prepared to retire and peter out.

Interest in sexual intercourse, according to Jennifer Hillman's findings, appeals to both sexes. So it would appear that older persons would be enjoying each others' company even more when Viagra is involved. Other studies, however, indicate conflicting responses. As discussed earlier, several women in the Potts et al. study took exception to their Viagra induced men by insisting that they had to participate in regular sexual intercourse. Worth noting is that the women from this study who found such frequency physically unpleasant were in the early middle to old age range. By contrast, Meika Loe's research of women older than the Potts et al. study group has shown that some widowed women have sought and found sexual satisfaction, while others have searched for such satisfaction and demanded that a female version of Viagra be made (Loe, 2004, pp. 310, 311). Maturity has made these women keen on "initiating" sexual relations. But their willingness often goes unrecognized and they have become marginalized, because their senior male counterparts' interests are directed not at them, but at much younger, sexually desirable women. It is as though the age of the men's sexual partners reflect how youthful and vigorous they perceive themselves. Loe has found that "Viagra (...) represents new sexual pressures sometimes leading to divorce and extramarital affairs [turning] husbands into sexualized animals (an 'old goat' and a 'frisky young colt'), leaving their wives frustrated and worn out" (Loe, 2004, pp. 313, 315; modification mine). Seeking other relations demonstrates that these men do not want to let go of their passions or let a sexual encounter go to waste. Even wasting a Viagra tablet is frowned upon by men (Potts et al., 2003, p. 704). So this seeking behavior leans towards excessiveness, because if one woman is worn out before the man is, surely a backup must lay in wait.

Age ceases to impair the "mad masters" when Viagra is involved. Diogenes may not have any notable issue with old people having sex, but the excessive lifestyle of the returning "mad masters" is one. As indicated earlier in his remark about lust, Diogenes prefers that people avoid being dominated by such an overactive appetite. Consider that Diogenes esteems some people when they do not give into their appetites. Diogenes Laertius confirms that Diogenes "was astonished that when slaves saw their masters were gluttons, they did not steal (...) viands" (D. L., 1991, p. 31). The irony here is that slaves are not slaves to their own appetitive masters, especially when the slaves, who may need food for the sake of survival, do not follow their masters' gluttonous lead. Although this anecdote is not of a sexual nature, it shows that Diogenes is impressed by those who can suppress their appetites. Remember he wished to stave off hunger by rubbing his belly as easily he could his sexual appetite through masturbation. *Askēsis*, or self-control, characterizes resoluteness in a person in spite of the appetite's strength. Those who fail to exercise *askēsis* are likely to face Diogenes' animadversion. Unfortunately there is no specific case of an elderly man engaged in excessive sexual activity in Diogenes' time—perhaps because Viagra was unavailable back then. But if one examines a modern situation where an old man takes Viagra for lots of sexual encounters with many women and compares that to Diogenes' response to those consumed by an excessive appetite, then an adequate account of how Diogenes would view the aged taking Viagra should materialize.

Given that most anecdotes present Diogenes confronting a person or small group of persons, we should focus on just one personal example of a man's excessive sexual debaucheries. In his research on foreigners travelling to China for the purpose of engaging in sexual liaisons with various Chinese women, James Farrer documents one incident involving an Australian man in his early sixties who is very sexually successful with several young women.

What stands out in this gentleman's own words is that he "provided them with good sex, he bragged, with the help of 'Viagra' tablets" (Farrer, 2010, p. 83). It is difficult from this confident admission to actually discern whether the old guy is a master lover or he has become a master due to his supplementary use of Viagra. Regardless of the reason, Viagra is an essential part of this man's ability to perform penetrative intercourse with so many different partners who tend to be around half or less than half his age. Without going into details about the social and socioeconomic factors behind the formation of such relations, the old man does not hide the fact that "sex was the main reason why he stayed in China" (Farrer, 2010, p. 83). This old man clearly has an almost unappeasable passion for sex. With so many available and willing partners, one wonders whether his carnal pleasure could possibly come to an end. Now if Diogenes could have encountered this particular individual, it is only fair to speculate on how unfavorable Diogenes' reaction would be of this man.

Relying on the anecdote where Diogenes criticizes a glutton of a man for being obese, one can get an idea as to how the philosopher would confront the sex crazed Australian pumped up on Viagra. Confronting a fat man for his excess, Diogenes announces, "'Let us beggars have something of your paunch; it will be a relief to you, and we shall get advantage'" (D. L., 1991, p. 59). This talk of relief and dispersal of excess through a distribution to those deprived is Diogenes' way of wanting the glutton to reduce his appetite to a healthy level that is fitting for a single person. To apply these lines of reasoning to one consumed by lust, one might think that Diogenes would beg the old man to have other single sex-starved men take turns with members of his harem, as it were. But these women are not viands and in conjunction with the philosopher's position on women consenting to sexual relations, they can decide on their own as to who penetrates them. Still, Diogenes would want to get the message across that this old man's fixation on sex and involvement with so many women is excessive. Rhetorically, Diogenes could request that the old guy give up on "good sex" by not taking Viagra. Would this brazen master be willing to give up the source of his stamina?

An affirmative response from Farrer's case study is unlikely, given his particular appetite. Factoring in Diogenes' wit, the old Australian businessman's own remarks about his sexual prowess in relation to his taking Viagra would be questioned, perhaps exposing who is truly behind these many exploits. Unlike Cephalus, the old man needs all the penile support he can get; otherwise, he to his disappointment may end up sexually destitute, or in other words, out of business. Those young willing Chinese women would then seek "good sex" from other masters. It may not be regarded as an ethical matter when a man partakes in so many liaisons, but Diogenes is interested in how an individual copes with one's appetite, which ultimately determines the kind of person he or she is. By adding Viagra to a very active libido, it appears that this old man seems to be coping very well and has no need of any relief. Even Diogenes admits that because of old age, he does not have to "slacken [his] pace" (D. L., 1991, p. 35; modification mine). An increase in one's pace should not, however, be compared to an increase in what an individual consumes. For Diogenes, the old man's appetite for sex has become twofold, in that he hungers for Viagra as much as he lusts after women. It is no longer a concern about sexual performance for the old man; instead, it has become a dependency problem.

Diogenes frequently regards lust as slavery (D. L., 1991, pp. 65, 69). Any man who admits that sex is the main reason why he remains in a particular state should be a concerning matter in terms of a personal vice. To develop an appetite for another item, viz., Viagra, on top of an existing appetite makes the Farrer's case study even more of a glutton. A life without Viagra in this particular example means a life without penetrative intercourse. Without calling this old man a sex and drug addict—which has become a problem among the sexual practices of various social groups (Lessenger et al., 2008, p. 49) –he has, by giving in to his appetite, voluntarily accustomed himself to a habitual lifestyle that has become compulsive. It is odd for this old man to discard women in much the same manner as Diogenes does away with material possessions he deems unnecessary burdens (D. L., 1991, p. 31). But unlike Diogenes, the old man quixotically continues to pursue women for sexual relations after his interest in his current relationship tends to wane. Ironically, because the old man's penis is now so full of life, the sexual relations with each of these young women cease to be fulfilling over time. Displaying no hard feelings towards the demise of these relationships, the old man maintains so-called friendships with most of them, especially his four ex-wives (Farrer, 2010, p. 83). In spite of the respect shown by the old man to his former lovers, his attitude about changing partners remains carefree, because his appetite is unchanged. As he grows older, the Australian will out of necessity always rely on his crutch—Viagra. For someone with this mindset, it would be preposterous to take into account Diogenes' reasoning that "the despising of pleasure is itself most pleasurable, when we are habituated to it…" (D. L., 1991, p. 73). To stop taking Viagra would additionally be preposterous for those whose passion for penetrative intercourse is incorrigible. Diogenes would not think highly of this old man for his indulgences, for the philosopher who favored the simple life held the view that "it was the privilege of the gods to need nothing and of god-like men to want but little" (D. L., 1991, p. 109). A lot less activity on the part of his penis might not make the old Australian a god-like man, but it might make him a little freer. Perhaps impotence is the best form of freedom from the "mad masters."

It is more of a challenge for any man to willingly minimize or eliminate his sexual appetites, especially when relations and the pleasures they produce are so readily available, than it is for him to cope with no sexual relations because of ED. Taking the little blue pill helps keep the carnal fountain of youth flowing. Diogenes prefers to see that men, young and old, defy their urges, avoid the temptations, and act in accordance with their age as in the case of youth studying philosophy and Didymon. This sentiment is most apparent when he gives advice on the appropriate time when a man should marry. He advises: "For a young man not yet: for an old man never at all" (D. L., 1991, p. 55). Although no precise age is ever given, Diogenes' point on time indicates that old men have expired and are likely unable to celebrate "'the bridal night.'" But if sexual urges according to Hillman and Llewellyn-Jones are natural in the aged, then why shouldn't the philosopher show some support for their using Viagra? Perhaps the extended length of time that Viagra keeps a penis erect would, by Diogenes' calculation, exceed its natural limitations. Viagra's effects on older men's penises ensure that they stay erect much longer than it ever did during the prime of their youth.

5. The Natural Death of the Penis: The Climax

An intriguing remark about the natural decline of penetrative intercourse comes from the Marquis de Sade's philosophical libertine, Dolmance. After introducing a young maiden to the joys of a variety of sexual acts, and upon discharging his build-up of sexual tension, he utters: "'tis done, I resist no longer…flow! my fluid flows!…and *I die*!…'" (Sade, 1990, p. 243; emphasis added). These words express a much more profound thought than just giving a detailed account of the climactic state of ejaculation during anal intercourse and the subsequent detumescence of the libertine's penis. Dolmance becomes fully aware that once his penis has performed all it can do, penetrative intercourse—whether it is anal, oral, or vaginal—is done. As lustful as Dolmance is, there is nothing in his power to keep it up. Additionally, the enjoyment of bodily pleasures no longer seems possible once his penis is incapable of being aroused, which may account for his extended break by giving a "stimulating" philosophical discussion about the nature of human passions before resuming further sexual lessons with the maiden. The part about dying suggests that there comes a time when penetrative intercourse and the pleasure it generates come to a conclusion, even though the desire for it remains. Many men would find this predicament, pun intended, a hard pill to swallow. It is then not difficult to see how hard pressed Dolmance or anyone like him would desire Viagra, since it "has a positive influence on the resumption of erection after ejaculation and has the potential to facilitate multiple instances of sexual intercourse in the presence of continuous erotic stimulus" (Aversa et al., 2000, p. 133). Eliminating the refractory period where men "are able to respond again to sexual stimuli and to re-enter the excitement phase" (Llewellyn-Jones, 1987, p. 93) and resisting the natural stage of resolution where the penis ceases to be aroused not only becomes crucial to prolonging sexual activity, it defies the natural flow of stimulation and arousal. Even the horniest of Sade's characters take the necessary time to rest before the next round of debauchery. So is the "positive influence" of Viagra an attempt to prevent the penis from dying?

Contrasting this point about the inevitable death of the penis to Diogenes' manner of thinking, one should return to how he commented on the eunuch's predicament. The eunuch's notable deficiency prevents him from penetrating any body cavity. He has reached a point in his life where the sexual activities that he was accustomed to are impossible. Diogenes recognizes that penetrative intercourse has reached its end for this particular man. Pfizer supported research, too, acknowledges that not all recipients of Viagra achieve youthful-like erections or the slightest stiffening of their muscles so as to partake in sexual intercourse (Dean et al., 2006, p. 781; Chevret-Méasson et al., 2009, p. 765). So when Diogenes questions how the eunuch is supposed to enter, especially after the quasi-epitaph forbidding entry to certain people has been erected, the eunuch does not take it to heart. Whether it is ignorance or denial, the eunuch, similar perhaps to some Viagra users or those longing to use the drug, cannot accept the reality of his handicap. Diogenes identifies this man by his apparent deficiencies—the inability to perform sexually and the inability to recognize his physical and moral limitations. Rhetorically, the penis and all it does determine a man's nature. In the case of the eunuch, he is nothing more than a prick, in spite of its absence. No wonder impotence is deemed by some men as a form of death (Marshall and Katz, 2002, p. 59; Potts et al., 2003, p. 706), for a lifeless penis takes the life out of a man with a still active sex drive.

Viewing impotence as death must make most men believe that Viagra is the best way to cheat it. Viagra keeps them alive through sexual activity. It is that which most, if not all, men live for. Sustaining this pharmaceutically enhanced lifestyle makes every man's life worth living. From that type of thinking, one recognizes how the blue pill can help immortalize the penis and its ongoing exploits. It subsequently appears as though the relationship between men and Viagra has become far more intimate than between a man and a woman.

Indifference characterizes Diogenes' limited treatment of death. There is nothing troubling about it, for "when in its presence we are not aware of it" (D. L., 1991, p. 69). Whatever dies is of no concern for the philosopher, for it has reached "a normal end to life" (Goulet-Cazé, 1996, p. 74). Consider how such thinking would apply to a man with an unresponsive penis. It is the underlying point Diogenes makes in the anecdote about the eunuch. The eunuch is not literally dead, but his sex life definitely is. Accepting one's fate reflects Diogenes' thoughts on the eunuch, especially when this specific death is involved. However, with Viagra's restorative powers and availability, impotent men, regardless of age, would most definitely defy such a fate.

Viagra now serves as a psychological crutch calming men's anxieties associated with their penises being or becoming lifeless. Expressed differently, there is a pharmaceutical prevention for the death of the penis and ultimately the sexual man. Restoring life can, in one sense, bring about fulfillment and excitement. For Diogenes, though, this relief signifies another kind of impotence, in that each man, out of fear, would consume Viagra so as to avoid his demise, albeit a synecdochical one. The philosopher who masturbated in public mentions another kind of slavery aside from lust; that is, "fear is the mark of the slave (...)" (D. L., 1991, p. 77). Once again, the notion of dependency applies to those who rely often on Viagra, for they fear impotency and Viagra is their convenient life-preserver. The more fearful a man is of his often softened penis the more vital it is for him to use the drug, especially when impotence is a fate worse than death (Marshall and Katz, 2002, p. 59). It is as though there is a longing for such men to be at the mercy of some mad master, and the pharmaceutical one will do just fine. As a social critic, Diogenes is not in the market to let this happen, because he excelled "in ruling men" (D. L. 1991, p. 77). This point illustrates his desire to guide, sometimes harshly, men to focus on more virtuous pursuits in life. Concentrating on the life of one's penis is a personal preoccupation that Diogenes would find very narcissistic, because that characteristic makes a man ignorant of other aspects of life aside from the life of his penis. Even Diogenes' eunuch carries on with life without being able to "enter" into domains of a penetrative nature.

Perhaps letting a man's penis expire naturally is the most fitting end. While Goulet-Cazé deduces what Diogenes' stance on religion may be, she offers an account as to how Diogenes developed an ability to cope with life's personal struggles. Her conclusion reads:

> Diogenes wants to be the master of his own destiny. The only limits to his freedom that he recognizes—because he cannot do otherwise—are the constraints imposed by nature. But in no way does he revere nature as one would a god. He simply has the wisdom not to struggle against it in vain. (Goulet-Cazé, 1996, pp. 79, 80)

Not devoid of personal struggle, Diogenes had put himself through various "hardships" (D. L. II, 1991, pp. 25, 27). This inuring of his body, another example of *askēsis*, toughens his character so as to accustom himself to extreme conditions. Preparing his body in thus manner enables him to endure the worst nature offers. So if Diogenes were to lose his erection, would he seek Viagra to remedy his loss? Given his remarks during his masturbatory episode, he would not find it any easier than to relieve his sexual appetite if his hands are free. If Viagra keeps a penis erect for such long periods of time, and if Diogenes were to take the drug (hypothetically speaking, of course), masturbation of a steadily erect penis, whether in public or not, might be too much of a burden for him to unload. If a god-like individual, mentioned earlier, should want little, Diogenes would give as little attention to his penis as possible. Giving no attention to Viagra would then ensure that he doesn't struggle against his own wisdom.

6. Conclusion: The Resolution

To attract the scorn of users, pushers, and makers of Viagra, Diogenes would only act consistent with how he always dealt with most people. Diogenes Laertius recounts that "[h]e was going into a theatre, meeting face to face, those who were coming out, and being asked why, [he answered that] 'this (...) is what I practice doing all my life'" (D. L. II, 1991, p. 67; modification mine). The confrontational approach is an appropriate response to those many individuals whom this philosopher criticized about their sexual practices, because there seems to be no inhibitions to what they practiced openly. Targeting prostitutes, effeminate men, those flaunting their assets, and profligates (D. L. II, 1991, pp. 39, 49, 53, 55, 61, 63, 65, 67, 69,) presents Diogenes as a man with a less than carefree attitude about human sexuality. Since Viagra impacts on human sexuality on a grand scale, both the user and those sexually involved with the user, Diogenes would animadvert individual users for not being "the master" of their respective actions. When Viagra restores the physiological part of the man, it becomes an issue as to who, or what, is in control of a sexually active penis.

The Pfizer ad mentioned in Simon-Maeda's article portrays the user as complacently possessed. It still is his desire, but there is something sinister behind what he can now do. Renewed confidence becomes inflated just like the erect penis. This intimate pairing of the psychological and physiological parts of a man then strives for one thing: penetrative intercourse. The man who has taken Viagra becomes mainly concerned with where his erect penis will take him. Entering into the world of recreational use of Viagra now contributes to a hedonistic and sometimes careless lifestyle that some men may find difficult to put to an end because of the pleasure intercourse produces and the revitalized ability to perform for the sake of such pleasure. For Diogenes, such men are slaves to their passions as well as the pharmaceutical aid which restores their sex lives. The derision Didymon receives from Diogenes for lusting after an unsuspecting young girl would correspondingly be directed at Farrer's old business man for sexually capitalizing on relations with several wives and young women. Regardless of the generations separating these men, the difference between them is that Viagra has transformed lust into gluttony. Viagra's convenience ensures that just as long as partners make themselves available a user can satisfy his seemingly endless appetite for much longer periods of time. There is a trade-off in keeping this sex drive alive, in that impotent men have no other option but to have Viagra back them up.

Looking closely at select anecdotes in Diogenes Laertius, one notices that curbing sexual desires and censuring specific sexual practices represent Diogenes' outlook on sexual relations. His frank offerings are not systematic, but they are consistent. The issues Viagra raises are of a sexual and moral nature, and since Diogenes frequently addresses sexual matters of the licentious and excessive kind, friction between the philosopher and most Viagra users would be inevitable. His seemingly conservative practice involving self-discipline (*askēsis*) and self-sufficiency (*autarkeia*) would rub viagrified lovers the wrong way. There simply is too much emphasis on sex and the penis for Diogenes to stomach. For instance, where is the discipline in the man who relies on Viagra for recreational fun? Discipline would interfere with the user's primal urge to enter into relations he so desires. But tell that to the women of the Potts et al. and Loe studies voicing distress and sometimes disdain at their partners' persistent eagerness and performance and believing viagrified sex consists of one-sided passion and is devoid of compassion. Viagra may enhance one part of an intimate relationship, but it does next to nothing for the overall relationship. Viagra users become easy targets for having an interest in immediate, carefree relations, because when looking at all of the sexually oriented anecdotes, one never finds Diogenes criticizing those who are in stable loving relations with women. Perhaps further study into his thoughts on human sexuality is required.

Returning to the point about being possessed by Viagra, one must come to realize that one body part that does not get enhanced is the rational part of man. Even though Viagra may boost a man's confidence in himself for being able to perform penetrative intercourse as before or possibly better, it does not excite his mind. The viagrified penis is in control. Sex becomes the sole purpose for a guy at that particular time, so there is nothing else for him to think about. Closing off one's mind so and putting so much attention on the penis and what it can do due to the drug's potency would make Diogenes think that such a man has not much to be proud of. Philosophically, when Diogenes strokes his penis in public, he is not stroking his ego. He offers insight into how different appetites are sated by different means. He has the upper hand over his appetite. Impotent men, on the other hand, consume Viagra so as to have their appetites consume them.

If Diogenes personally had to handle impotency, would he be as relieved as Cephalus when the "mad masters" no longer trouble him? Or to ask a second time, would he relish the opportunity to be born anew by taking Viagra? Given how Diogenes cared for himself, his response to the last question would be identical to the one he gave while dining at a temple. According to the anecdote, "in the course of the meal loaves not free from dirt were put on the table, he took them up and threw them away, declaring that *nothing unclean ought to enter* a temple" (D. L. II, 1991, p. 65; emphasis added). Opting not to consume that which is unsavory reveals how Diogenes is not in the market of corrupting his body or his mind. So to respond to the initial question pertaining to the influence of the "mad masters," Diogenes would not be perturbed if his sexual appetite passed away, for it is one less appetite for him to sate. If impotency is equated with death, Diogenes would not fear ED. Perhaps a modernized anecdote of Diogenes encountering a man taking Viagra so as to indulge in penetrative intercourse would have the philosopher question the user as such: When your penis has run its course and has withered and died, why make it hard for yourself by raising it from the dead?

Notes

1. "In 1983, Dr Giles Brindley astounded an audience of his colleagues at a conference by injecting his penis with phenoxybenzamine and displaying, for all to see, an erection obtained by purely chemical means" (Marshall and Katz, 2002, p. 54). The similarity between Dr Brindley and Diogenes is not how they achieved their erections, but how they had no inhibitions at publicly exposing their penises in order to make a point. With the philosopher, however, his erection arose without medicinal assistance.
2. Not fully certain is whether the two accounts of Diogenes' masturbatory episode in Diogenes Laertius and the one Galen recounts are related. Given the lack of specific details, it is unlikely so. The reason being is that since the two glib accounts in Diogenes Laertius are identical and take place in a public setting, it is only conceivable that a courtesan may have been present among the crowd when Diogenes was masturbating. Besides, the courtesan is a prominent figure in Galen's account, not Diogenes Laertius'. Galen does not even claim that the event was done in public and there is no mention of Diogenes' remark about hunger or his belly. Perhaps Diogenes often struggled with this desire to stimulate his penis, so when it became too much for him to handle, other persons happen to be around to witness this struggle with himself. Not many with a scholarly or a philosophical disposition desire to investigate Diogenes' masturbatory episode to any great extent beyond the notion of *autarkeia*.
3. Almost all of the interpretations of this anecdote, which lack significant development, portray Diogenes as one who would amass women for the purpose of sexual intercourse (Rist, 1969, p. 60; Long, 1996, p. 42; Billerbeck, 1996, pp. 210, 211; Schofield, 1999, pp. 12, 125). However, the formation of such a community rests on a woman's consent. Note the singular reference. Without mutual desire and interest, there is no reason for any freethinking woman to enter into such relations, unless she knowingly or willingly wants to.

Three

A QUESTION OF VIRTUOUS SEX: WOULD ARISTOTLE TAKE VIAGRA?

Thomas Kapper

1. Introduction

While the hypothetical title query is perhaps somewhat glib, it does intimate the non-hypothetical, "should *anyone* take Viagra?" This essay will apply Aristotelian ethics to that question, specifically whether the typical user's, "It makes me happy" rationale withstands critical scrutiny. In addition, we examine whether sex with the aid of Viagra can be considered natural and relate this to the ancient notion, via Stoic philosophy, that the life lived best is one in harmony with what occurs by nature.

The thought of Aristotle has been selected for this task, but how can a Greek philosopher born in 384 B.C.E. have anything worthwhile to say about such a contemporary issue? Present-day philosophical thinking and writing appear to bypass, at least to the casual observer, questions that really matter. What should we do? What is a meaningful life to lead? Unlike much of the philosophy found in today's academy where the writing seems to be for other academics of similar sub-specialties and impenetrable to the general public, the ancients (admittedly a generalization but true of Aristotle) had a practical goal, to help students to become good, or better, people. Philosophy was life itself and more than simply a day job. Current Western philosophy seems to be merely a branch of knowledge like biology or botany, and the philosopher a person "who goes through particular doctrines during his courses but, once he goes home, lives exactly like his lawyer or his dentist without what he teaches having the slightest influence on the way he lives his life" (Revel and Ricard, 1998, p. 101). Even so, certainly any number of ethical systems could be applied to the Viagra issue. Why turn to the ancients in general and Aristotle in particular?

Aristotle had a singular focus on the good life, on what is the best way to live. His ethics are not just a general treatise on the nature of that life but rather are practical guidelines for the achievement of such an existence. The root of what brings us to Aristotle is his emphasis on the social. He notes that it is a human inclination to live in the company of others, and the truly good life is only possible with mutuality. This mutuality "is a virtue, or involves virtue, and besides is most necessary for our life. For no one would choose to live without friends even if he had all other goods" (1155a1-5).[1] Thus, if we combine the fact that Viagra is an eminently as well as intimately social drug with the near truism that sexual function has become central to contemporary conceptions of the good life, then engaging the thought of Aristotle promises to be fruitful.

2. Aristotle's Ethics

From the ancients[2] we have the beginnings of philosophy in the West and with it the perpetually daunting questions of just what comprises the good life and just how is it to be achieved. Aristotle was not the first to take up these issues, but he was the first to write systematically on ethics as a distinct topic, not unexpected for the consummate overachiever. He was a student of Plato and made seminal contributions to almost every field of knowledge. His physics lasted until the seventeenth century, his biology until Darwin, and his logic until the late nineteenth century.[3] His ethical system is arguably the longest lived, having enjoyed something of a resurgence in the second half of the twentieth century (MacIntyre, 1984).

The source of Aristotle's thought for this essay is the *Nicomachean Ethics* written about 350 B.C.E. It can be viewed as his work on politics from the point of view of the individual. The Ethics is not an easy treatise. It is dense with ideas and lacks the poetic verve of a Plato. The language is terse almost to the point of being considered lecture notes. It "has a dry conciseness that makes one imagine one is perusing a table of contents rather than a book; it tastes for all the world like chopped hay" (Quennell, 1988, p. 168). It is filled with winding arguments and digressions to be sure but also repays reading with perspicuous insights.

The Ethics lays out Aristotle's vision of what can be termed virtue ethics. Virtue ethics focuses on the composition of character, on which dispositions are morally good (virtues), rather than on rules that determine which action is good or right. Simply put, a good person will do the right thing. Virtue is the traditional translation of the Greek word *arête*. This is also sometimes translated as "excellence" and in the ethical realm it refers primarily to matters of character. A virtue is a character trait that humans, given their physical and psychological nature, need in order to flourish, or to do and fare well (Statman, 1996). For Aristotle, this was acting and feeling according to reason, choosing a mean between the opposite flaws of excess and deficiency, finding an appropriate response for whatever situation presents itself. But Aristotle notes that virtue is no undemanding end to attain.

> Hence it is hard work to be excellent, since in each case it is hard work to find what is intermediate; e.g. not everyone, but only one who knows, finds the midpoint in a circle. So also getting angry, or giving and spending money, is easy and anyone can do it; but doing it to the right person, in the right amount, at the right time, for the right end, and in the right

> way is no longer easy, nor can everyone do it. Hence, doing these things well is rare, praiseworthy and fine (1109a25-30).

The methodology was the same with those stirrings recognized as passions; the key was to find the ideal compromise between too much and too little of any emotion. For example, bodily pleasures are fine in moderation; it is only excessive indulgence that is damaging. "Some sources of pleasure are necessary; others are choice-worthy in themselves, but can be taken to excess" (1147b25).

An issue to be addressed early on in the current essay is its largely sexual subject matter. It is a topic (under the guise of *Eros*) that Aristotle, unlike his teacher Plato, spilled very little ink over. However, Books VIII and IX of the Ethics deal with Friendship.[4] In fact, no other single topic in the Ethics is dealt with at a similar length. Friendship is a translation of the Greek term *philia* which is a somewhat more plastic term than "friend." For our purposes we will interpret *friendship* as the broader term *relationship* and see what insights that can gain for us (that sound you hear are scholars of Aristotle simultaneously slapping their foreheads).[5] From relationships in general we can move the discussion to sexual relationships.

While Aristotle claimed that one can specify certain virtues that are necessary to cultivate to live a good life, sex (or to use the noun form, sexiness or sexual desirability) was not among them. Nor was sex mentioned as a path to a virtuous life (which is somewhat disappointing). Rather virtuous sex can only be construed as sexual activity engaged in by the good person. And the partner of that good person is a friend indeed.

Now to begin. The bearded and robed philosopher holds a blue pill up to the light and says, "But what is it?"

3. Does Taking Viagra Really Make You Happy?

We begin with a useful analogy. In earlier times, hunting for food, whether wildlife or ripe fruits, was solely for the purpose of sustenance, a necessity for survival. In today's world hunting, more often than not, is referred to as "sport." Similarly, the clinical and market success of Viagra appears to have moved the understanding of sexual function in the male entirely outside of reproductive concerns (Kaiser, 1999, p. 44). Viagra is the prototype of a group of medications that treat what until recently were conditions considered to be the natural result of aging or within the normal range of healthy human functioning, e.g. male pattern baldness, shyness, too thin eyelashes. These are lifestyle drugs, and a chief characteristic of the medicalization of ordinary life (Loe, 2006). "So what," says the typical user. "Taking Viagra makes me happy." To which the dubious philosopher replies, "Are you certain?"

In the Ethics, Aristotle speaks of a good that we seek for its own sake and no other reason. The possession of that good will leave us in need of nothing; it is the complete and self-sufficient good and not a means to some other good.

> Suppose, then, that there is some end of things we pursue in our actions which we wish for because of itself, and because of which we wish for the other things; and we do not choose everything because of something else, since if we do, it will go on without limit, making desire empty and futile; then clearly this end will be the good, the best good" (1094a18-22).

This good Aristotle called Happiness. Rather that is what many of his translators have called it. Aristotle himself used the term *eudaimonia*. Eudaimonia has been called a term that is difficult to spell, pronounce, and understand, often at the same time (Ryff and Singer, 2006), a criticism not without merit. One problem with its direct translation as happiness is that doing so equates hedonia, pleasure or pleasant feeling, with eudaimonia, something very much at odds with Aristotle's ideas. A closer rendering of eudaimonia is human flourishing, a more expansive notion. Our contemporary view of happiness is generally synonymous with hedonia, but eudaimonia applies to a whole life and its rootedness rather than merely what it feels like. The modern concept of happiness is thin compared with eudaimonia.

In fact, Aristotle is uneasy about pleasure. At one point, he disparagingly refers to the pursuit of pleasure as a "life for grazing animals" (1095b20). Yet he spends a great deal of time in Book X explaining, in a not fully satisfying way, just why hedonism is not the greatest good. At the risk of oversimplifying, Aristotle concludes that the best life will indeed be pleasant, but pleasure alone is an uncertain guide to the good life. As the contemporary philosopher Robert Nozick puts it, "there is more to life than being happy" (Nozick, 1989, p. 106).

Thus our typical Viagra user, suitably schooled by Aristotle, restates his position, "Taking Viagra gives me pleasure." But the skeptic quickly responds, "Not so fast." It is not Viagra that causes the pleasure. The pill allows/enhances a resultant sexual experience. Thus, it differs from Prozac, cocaine, etc. all of which have a direct effect in the user's brain. It is not as simple as spending the weekend prostrate in an opium den. A successful Viagra result requires further action, and as mentioned, that action ideally requires a partner.

There are three aspects of sexual pleasure that Viagra seeks to enhance. The first is pure physical sensation. Here sex serves as a reminder that humans are animals; in the end we are just clever apes that speak. Sex, as stated in characteristic Stoic fashion by the Roman Emperor Marcus Aurelius, is a "friction of the members and an ejaculatory discharge" (quoted in Irvine, 2009, p. 139). This first can be classified as biological.

The second aspect deals more with the mind. Sex results in an ego stroking ranging from machismo and an effusive swagger to a simple increased confidence. This is the psychological realm. The third is being with and sharing something, with a partner. While we hesitate to call this 'spiritual' (that is better left to the poets), the fullness of a sexual relationship is certainly social. Here we can begin to expand Aristotle's ideas of friendship.

4. It Takes Two to Tango: Aristotle, Friendship, and Sex

To this point, our title query can be restated thus: Can taking Viagra harm a relationship by decreasing the user's virtue while ostensibly making him happy (pleasure not eudaimonia) and consequently side-tracking his path to the truly good life? The next step in pursuing this now quite wordy question, is to turn to Aristotle and his thinking on friendships. As mentioned, he is concerned with more than what we would consider friendship proper. His concern, on our reading, is with broader relationships.

In the Ethics, Aristotle's treatment of friendships falls into roughly three areas. For our purposes we are only concerned with the first, his classification scheme of friendships. He enumerates three, grouped by their different forms and purposes. The first is friendship of utility. "Those who love each other for utility love the other not in himself, but in so far as they gain some good for themselves from him" (1156a11-12). As could be surmised, this is a friendship based on usefulness. Here we can see relationships in commerce, such as the small talk made with a bartender. In addition, this is the friendship found frequently among co-workers. Whether a friendship is one of utility or pleasure, Aristotle's second category, can be determined by considering whether you hang out with work friends *after* work as well.

A sexual friendship of utility is perhaps most clearly exemplified by prostitution. While this is not Aristotle's example he makes some prescient points about this type of friendship:

> Nor do such people live together very much. For sometimes they do not even find each other pleasant. Hence they have no further need to meet in this way if they are not advantageous to each other; for each finds the other pleasant only to the extent that he expects some good from him (1156a28-32).

Each side profits; one by sensual sensation the other by monetary remuneration. Adding Viagra to this relationship changes little. Both partners have every reason to expect satisfaction from increasing the frequency of the encounters. It would be an interesting investigation to explore whether the introduction of Viagra increases the prevalence of prostitution. The possibility cannot be fully discounted. There is also a more subtle form of the notion of this sexual utility. Women in some relationships trade sex for gifts, favors, etc.

Although in fact this may not be done consciously, it is utility just the same and again Viagra is most likely a boon.

In modern terms, a friendship of utility is referred to as an acquaintance. 'Friendships of pleasure' is how most of us would construe the majority of our own friendships. Pleasure refers to mutual pleasure, as seen from each partner's own point of view. A prime example is friends having a drink or simply hanging out. Aristotle says that we "like a witty person not because of his character, but because he is pleasant" (1156a13) to be around. The object too of a sexual friendship based on pleasure is for the sake of pleasure to oneself. This is exemplified in the youthful notion of "hooking up" or for a slightly older generation the "one night stand." Again Aristotle is prescient on these matters: "Young people are prone to erotic passion, since this mostly follows feelings, and is caused by pleasure; that is why they love and quickly stop, often changing in a single day" (1156b2-4). Again the addition of Viagra is not a detriment but rather may increase the likelihood of such encounters.

Aristotle's third type of friendship is one grounded in virtue. This is labeled with the Greek term *teleia philia* which is usually translated as "completed" or "perfected" friendship. It is a friendship of excellence or character. Teleia is etymologically related to telos, the goal or end of something. The adjective teleios often qualifies its noun as something "fully developed." In describing a friendship in this fashion, one would mean not just the fully developed form of friendship, but a development that completes the intended purpose of the thing. Thus, we can see the grounding of this form of friendship as virtue itself.

It is a friendship of a profoundly moral nature. One wants what is best for one's friend for the friend's sake. It is fully selfless. Each friend helps the other to fully realize his or her own virtue. For Aristotle these are the friendships of a lifetime. There is some similarity to the other friendships. "Friendship for pleasure bears some resemblance to this complete sort, since good people are also pleasant to each other. And friendship for utility also resembles it, since good people are also useful to each other" (1157a1-3).

A sexual relationship of the perfected type could be an ideal successful marriage or other long-term relationship. It is into this type of relationship that the introduction of Viagra can be problematic. Viagra can provoke selfishness in the male, an overemphasis on the first two aspects of pleasure. The raw sensuality can blind him to the wants and needs of his partner.[6] The same can be said of the increased ego stroking. There is a tendency for the social aspect, the partner's needs and vital role, to be severely downplayed or overlooked altogether.

The most optimal situation would fully integrate Viagra into the relationship. The couple would remain in the perfect friendship with the Viagra-enhanced sex becoming just another aspect of the relationship. The danger is in regressing to lesser friendships. Here we note that Aristotle's friendships are not a hierarchy, but a classification. A friendship does not progress up through them to attain the rarified perfection. Thus to say regress is not fully accurate. Even so, the perfect friendship is at the top, and any change would be going to something less, which is by definition a regression.

A change to a friendship of pleasure would be the next best thing. The worst case is that Viagra may change the sexual relationship to one of utility. For example, the male gets sensual pleasure while the female achieves peace in the household. In sexual friendships of utility and pleasure, there is a risk of viewing, and using, other people merely as interesting sensations. This reflects a certain shallowness and these relationships are often short-lived. For pleasure, the sexual attraction may whither. The friendship only survives as long as the sensual pleasure does. "When the beloved's bloom is fading, sometimes the friendship fades too; for the lover no longer finds pleasure in seeing his beloved, while the beloved is no longer courted by the lover" (1157a8-10). For even with Viagra, there must at least be a tiny spark of desire. For utility, well, in the prostitution example one may run short of funds. "Those who are friends for utility dissolve the friendship as soon as the advantage is removed; for they were never friends of each other, but of what was expedient for them" (1157a15).

The first two friendships are more centered on the self while the third emphasizes the well-being of the other. This, according to Aristotle, is because you so admire your companion's virtue. One of the interesting synonyms of virtue, and one not unrelated to the current topic, is chastity. This meaning has obvious Victorian roots and overtones, and to risk one's virtue was a serious matter indeed. In a similar way, to risk the perfect friendship, the friendship of virtue, with the use of Viagra is also serious, and requires the same thoughtful consideration.

5. Stoicism, Viagra, and the Natural Lifecourse

Men at forty
Learn to close softly
The doors to rooms they will not be
Coming back to.
Donald Justice, 'Men at Forty'

We now turn to a second school of ancient thought, the Stoics. Would the true Stoic use Viagra? Absolutely not. Sex was filled with pitfalls, emotional and sensual, which run counter to sought after tranquility. However, our interest is in the Stoic notions of the naturalness of life, duty, and fate.

The Stoics disagreed with Aristotle on many if not most issues. Yet they shared a concern with what comprises a life well-lived. As the philosopher Lawrence C. Becker puts it, "Stoic ethics is a species of eudaimonism. Its central, organizing concern is about what we ought to do or be to live well—to flourish" (Becker, 1998, p. 20). The Stoics were active across a span of half a millennium in antiquity and their theories were revived in early modernity and have persevered to our time. Three more or less distinct Stoic schools stretch over the five hundred years. The Early Stoa began about 300 B.C.E. in Athens. It was named after the venue where the Stoics taught, the painted portico (*stoa poikile*) in the Athenian marketplace. Zeno of Citium, the founder, enjoyed the portico because he preferred to pace up and down while teaching.[7] We do not have extended works by Zeno, but only fragments preserved by later writers. Thus the philosophical framework comes to us piecemeal.

The Middle Stoa lasted to the end of the first century B.C.E. It was in this phase that Stoicism began to become more of a movement. The doctrines began to pervade the Roman governing and military classes. Cicero's *Tusculan Disputations* (45 B.C.E.) is the most accessible account of the first two Stoic schools.

The last phase, the Late Stoa, ran to roughly 200 C.E. It was largely ethically oriented. The slave Epictetus and the emperor Marcus Aurelius wrote in this spirit. As a philosophical school Stoicism faded, but as a movement it went popular.[8] It was an attitude in tune with a precarious world.

Zeno believed that happiness should be based on reason, not pleasure. He insisted that the wise man was not free to ignore his duties and obligations to others. Living the good life meant engaging with society. This social involvement echoed Aristotle. The concern for others made the good life less than serene, entailing the messy, often disordered circumstances of human lives. Thus, there arose the ideal of *apatheia*, apathy, no emotional or passionate indulgence. The Stoic theory of the passions in a nutshell is that emotions are mistakes. Every passion is an impulse which is disobedient to reason. The passions are pathological, a sickness, the sickness of letting a pathos overcome a logos. Stoicism spares no time to dwell on moods or wallow in feelings.

We should strive to be better people, to become virtuous in the ancient sense. For the Stoics, virtue depends on one's excellence as a human being—on how well you perform the functions for which humans were designed. As Zeno put it, this is to live in accordance with nature. If we do this, we have a good life. The Stoic finds virtue in cultivating the naturalness of life and in the roles one plays and the duties one has across the lifecourse. According to Cicero, philosophy helps us to live according to nature at every stage of life; the natural life has but a single course that every human must move through, and we must adapt to each of life's stages appropriately. Aging is a question of character.

Epictetus states that we should keep firmly in mind that we are merely actors in a play written by someone else. We cannot choose our role, but regardless of the role chosen for us, we must do our utmost. Marcus also advocates taking a fatalistic attitude toward life. To do otherwise is to rebel against nature, and such rebellions are counterproductive, if what we seek is a good life. We must learn to adapt ourselves to the environment into which fate has placed us (Irvine, 2009). In this context of naturalness, the Stoic Seneca praises the slackening of desire that accompanies age, "How comforting it is to have tired out one's appetites, and to have done with them!" (quoted in Irvine, 2009, p. 193).

Even into the twentieth century, it was strongly held that sexual decline follows naturally in tandem with growing older and coping with it is part of the basic moral exercise of adjustment to the effects of the aging process (Haber, 1983). Advice from the year 1900 states that with impotence there is no remedy and one should submit as gracefully as possible to the decrees of fate (Sturgis, 1900). However, one gets the sense of making the best of a bad situation; the sighing is nearly palpable. The language sounds a great deal like a rationalization: "The stress of passion will be past, the imagination will become more chastened, the heart more refined, the lines of intellectual and spiritual vision lengthened, the sphere of usefulness enlarged" (Stall, 1901, p. 59). Aging "is calmly welcomed by many as a release from turmoil, permitting greater and deeper enjoyment of other beauties of living" (Stieglitz, 1949, p. 197). There seems to be an undercurrent of grasping. The fact is that most older adults report moderate or high levels of sexual interest well into their 70's (DeLamater and Sill, 2005).

Is it desire that deserts the body? Or is the spirit willing but the flesh weak? A recent generation has responded that the spirit is indeed willing. Members of the baby boom generation are said to have venerated youth until it became their social value, and have stubbornly gripped to it even as they have aged. In the late twentieth century, gerontology had determined that sexual activity, particularly sexual intercourse, was a healthy and necessary component of successful aging. Age without sex was literally old-fashioned (Katz and Marshall, 2003). The contemporary attitude is "you don't stop having sex because you get old, you get old because you stop having sex" (Danoff, 1993, p. 156).

The rules are being rewritten. The Stoic response is reconfigured for Viagra. Zeno and Cicero may be correct that the ideal life follows nature, but who decides whether Viagra is natural? Katz and Marshall (2004) have stated that with Viagra, there is "no pretense of a natural body." But in a nation of nose jobs and breast implants, no one is tied to the wonders of what is arbitrarily decreed natural. An obvious version of the doctrine of naturalism holds that if something exists in the physical world, it is natural. Nature is all there is. Claims that Viagra is not natural betrays a clinging to tradition and cultural norms.

When you think about it, of the various philosophical schools, Stoicism can be considered the winner. For when people speak of "being philosophical about it," they mean "taking it stoically." They have in mind a version of life devised to gain personal control in a large, hazardous world, a way of life strenuously concentrated on subjective, inward control. It is to determinedly let go of whatever is not "up to us"—which is everything external. A Stoic may decline Viagra, but not because it is not natural but rather because it hinders *apatheia*. From the Stoic perspective, the virtuous sex is often the sex which does not happen at all.

Viagra seeks whatever spark of desire is there and fans it into a flame. As Dylan Thomas said, "rage against the dying of the light." The youth-obsessed West in the 21st century will not go gentle into that good night.

5. Conclusion: Viagra and Fullness of Fate

From an Aristotelian perspective, there is moral risk in the use of Viagra. Without approaching its use with one's eyes wide open, aware of the potential pitfalls, certainly relationships can be harmed. A relationship based in virtue can dissolve. The problem stems from a failure to fully address the needs and desires of the partner. The question of what women want has become a cliché due to the frequency of the asking. It is raised at regular intervals in the cycling cultural zeitgeist. The answer from men this time around is Viagra. The answer from women goes unheard due to the shattering volume of the male response.

Consider, for example, a widespread series of television commercials. The voiceover says something to the effect of "when the time is right" and shows a couple, middle-aged, making eyes at each other. In viewing the spot, women read into it love while men read into it sex. Potts is explicit in encapsulating the problem: "More attention needs to be paid to partners' perspectives and desires, and to the specific dynamics of any given relationship" (Potts et al., 2003, p. 697).

Perhaps Viagra delays the fullness of one's fate, the full maturation of the individual praised by the Stoics. A cynic would say that Viagra conspires in a prolonging of adolescence to absolute absurdity. Marcus Aurelius advocates loving ones fate if indeed one seeks a good life. But then again, just as Viagra may be considered natural so too may it be part of one's fate. In Greek mythology, the goddess Ananke was the personification of destiny, necessity, and fate itself. Ananke gradually fell out of favor and was replaced by none other than Eros, god of sexual desire. Perhaps the ancients would have understood Viagra all too well.

As for the title query, would Aristotle himself take Viagra? One could speculate that he of all people would recognize the possibility of jeopardizing that perfect mutuality that so contributes to the good life. In the end, though, he was the son of a physician and a quarter of his surviving works do deal with biology (a fascination with cuttlefish to be sure). One has to believe that his curiosity would win out.

Notes

1. References to Aristotle are to the Terence Irwin translation of the *Nicomachean Ethics* and are annotated with standard Bekker numbers.

2. For the dates for ancient philosophy, we will somewhat arbitrarily assign the dates from the 7th century B.C.E. to the end of the Roman Empire in the 4th century C.E.
3. Here are two additional interesting Aristotelian facts. He was a tutor to Alexander the Great. In the late Middle Ages, he was referred to simply as The Philosopher.
4. The *Nichomachean Ethics* is broken into ten Books, what in contemporary writing we would refer to as chapters.
5. Aristotle's friendships explicitly omit women from the discussion, but we need not adhere to this stricture. He was in many ways a product of his time.
6. This is unfortunately true of many males *not* using Viagra as well.
7. As an interesting parallel, adherents of Aristotle's school were known as Peripatetics, perhaps because of their teacher's reported habit of strolling while conversing.
8. The temptation was to use the phrase "went *viral*" thus thoroughly dating the current essay to 2010.

Four

MAN'S FALLEN STATE: ST. AUGUSTINE ON VIAGRA

Kevin Guilfoy

> But even those who delight in sexual pleasure are not moved to it at their own will, whether they confine themselves to lawful, or transgress to unlawful pleasures; but sometimes this lust importunes them in spite of themselves, and sometimes fails them when they desire to feel it, so that though lust rages in the mind, it stirs not in the body. Thus, strangely enough, this emotion not only fails to obey the legitimate desire to beget offspring, but also refuses to serve lascivious lust; and though it often opposes its whole combined energy to the soul that resists it, sometimes also it is divided against itself, and while it moves the soul, leaves the body unmoved. (*City of God* 14.16)

1. Introduction

Lust, or concupiscence, is one of the punishments for original sin. In our fallen state we do not have voluntary control over our own desires and we do not have voluntary control over our own genitals. Like all young men Augustine was perhaps too aware of half of the problem. Lust rages in our minds and we cannot make it stop. This lust can "move the body" at inconvenient times, much against our will. We want the lust to be gone, and we want control over our bodies. But as this passage from the *City of God* shows, the older more mature Augustine saw the other half of the problem. Sometimes we want the lust but we cannot make ourselves feel the desire, and sometimes when we feel the desire the body remains unmoved. We do not have voluntary control over our sexual desires, and we do not have voluntary control over the organs we would use to act on those desires. Erectile dysfunction is the result of man's fallen state. If Viagra works as advertised it gives men partial voluntary control over their sexual desires and their genitals. While this may approximate our perfect pre-fall state, Augustine would still find Viagra artificial and problematic.

It may seem a moot point to explore Augustine's thoughts on Viagra. In the west impressions of Christian negativity towards sex are common. Some of these impressions are exaggerated caricatures. Some are not. Many owe their origin to Augustine (Miles, 2005, p. 322; Brown, 1988). According to Augustine humans suffer from a disordered and culpable lust that infects all post-fall human sexual relations. This is our punishment for original sin, and it is the basis of centuries of ethical teachings that made us ashamed of our sexual desires. Even if one is not one of the millions of people who live explicitly according to (current interpretations) of Augustine's teachings, in the west, we all live in a culture shaped by Augustine's ideas. If you are reading this book with a furtive and prurient sense of secrecy, then you owe some of that sense of shame to St. Augustine.[1]

Augustine's earliest writings on sex are quite stridently opposed to it. For better or worse these early writings have exerted the most cultural influence and shaped the received view of Augustine's thought (Miles, 2005; Burke, 1990; Hunter, 1994). Throughout his career he maintained that we should all strive to be free of lustful sexual desire, and if we cannot be free of the desire we should still try to be strong enough to abstain. But as he aged, Augustine came to understand that the expression of sexual love in marriage is the foundation of a deep and meaningful bond between husband and wife. Marriage is a lesser good than chastity, but a faithful, sexually-active marriage is a genuine good. It is in this context that Viagra presents an interesting problem for Augustine. Viagra is a tool that helps men to have sex. Men take Viagra thinking that it can boost their libido creating stronger desire for sex and give them the ability to act on the desire.[2] Obviously Viagra will not help a man to achieve the higher good of chastity. Equally obviously this tool can be used to achieve the evils of adultery or fornication. So it would seem that Augustine's thoughts on Viagra might be clear. If Viagra cannot help a person achieve the highest good, and can be used to do evil, then Viagra should not be used.

On the other hand, a faithful, sexually-active marriage is a genuine good. It seems that a couple could use Viagra, with the proper intentions to achieve the lower goods of procreation and marital friendship. Lower goods are those that by definition can be sought excessively, too much of them can harm a person. In the trite formulation of an intro philosophy class: food is good, too much food is harmful; love of God is a higher good, and there is no such thing as too much love of God. It is always risky to seek lower goods, and precarious to attain them. There are, I think, a few circumstances where an older mature Augustine would give a heavily qualified and always tentative endorsement of Viagra as a tool to seek and obtain the lower goods of marriage.

2. Augustine's Early Opposition to Sex

Augustine's earliest thoughts on sex and marriage developed in his personal conversion struggle. He understood his conversion as a turning away from sexual lust and a turning to Christianity. In the *Soliloquies* (386ce) and the dialogues of the Casiacum period (386–387ce), a 32 year old, and obviously emotionally young, Augustine writes of his struggles with unbridled sexual desire. These earliest ideas on sex and marriage reflect a naïve Platonism and some remaining vestiges of Manichean thought. Augustine asserts that "nothing brings the manly mind down from the heights like a woman's caresses and the joining of bodies." He resolves "not to covet, not to seek and not to marry a wife!" (Sol. I.10.17). Like many young men, he thinks of marriage and women only in the terms of sexual desire. For the young Augustine, sexual desire is a shameful distraction from higher truth and spirituality. The *Soliloquies*, despite the title, are a dialogue between Augustine and a personification of Reason. Upon hearing Augustine's assertion, Reason asks him whether he still experiences desire and lust. Augustine says that he does not. Reason presses the point; the next day Reason asks Augustine about his thoughts as he lay in bed last night. "While lying awake (…) you realized how, differently from your claims, those imagined caresses and bitter sweetnesses still excited you" (Sol. I.14.25). He cannot control himself yet, but Augustine believes that a person can and should voluntarily control both his actions and his desires. Abstaining from sex is an act of will, but so is refraining from the desire for sex. This belief that the person, by force of will, ought to exert voluntary control not just over his body but also over his desires is more fully developed in *On Free Choice of the Will* (386ce). He writes that if your will is subject to passions and desire that dictate your choices: "Your servitude is your own fault and your unhappiness is just; since you could overpower this thing if you willed to do so" (FCW 3.6). Our desires should not be dictating our choices. Instead our desires themselves should be in our voluntary control. We should be able to choose which desires we experience.

When he writes his autobiography, the *Confessions*, in 397ce at the age of 43, he still believes that he can make himself desire what he ought to desire. He believes he can make himself want chastity. Augustine at age 43 looks back on his sexual past and recognizes that he knew what he ought to want. He ought to want chastity. He even wanted to want chastity. He just did not have the strength of will to actually want chastity. Thus at age 43 he describes the prayer of a young man: "God grant me chastity and continence, but not yet" (Conf. 8.7.17).

Describing his conversion Augustine is explicit about his sexual lust and how this kept his from embracing Christianity.

> My ancient mistresses, still held me; they plucked my fleshy garment, and whispered softly, (…) what did they suggest, O my God? Let Thy mercy turn it away from the soul of Thy servant. What defilements did they suggest! What shame! And now I much less than half heard them.

But then Continence personified appears:

> her holy hands full of multitudes of good examples: there were so many young men and maidens here, a multitude of youth and every age, grave

> widows and aged virgins. (…) And she smiled on me with a persuasive mockery, as would she say, "Canst not thou do what these youths, what these maidens can?" (Conf. 8.11.15)

Augustine then walks into the garden where he has his famous moment of conversion. At the time he was writing the Confessions, Augustine still believed that upon true conversion to Christianity one gained the strength of will to become chaste in thought and deed.

Augustine's early view is perhaps not the healthiest understanding of human sexuality, and obviously leaves no room for a licet use of Viagra. But as this early view has had great influence it is worth outlining the argument. For a man with strong sexual desire but erectile dysfunction Viagra is just another step in the procurement of sex. Such a man is already distracted by desire. Without Viagra, this first man might eventually turn to more spiritual pursuits, but this is unlikely.

> The man, however, who yields to lust a wicked service, receives such great energies that, even when all his members are now failing through age, and those special parts of his body are unable to be applied to their proper function, he does not ever cease to revel in a still increasing rage of disgraceful and shameless desire. (MC 1.28)

Viagra is simply enabling this first man to consummate the sins he is already consenting to in his mind. His actions are culpable but easily understood.

A second man who takes Viagra because he has lost the desire for sex is a far more troubling case for Augustine. This second man finds himself with low libido or diminished sex drive. He has, without any effort, achieved the absence of desire that Augustine believed he could achieve with his conversion. The second man's choice to use Viagra represents a truly inverted value system. This man finds himself at greater liberty to seek higher spiritual goods and chooses to create the desire for lower sexual goods. This man is not a slave to sexual desire. This man is a slave to the desire for sexual desire. This second man wants to want what he surely knows he ought not to want. He values sex and wants to want sex. This represents a much graver moral error.

The human ability to knowingly seek lower goods, at the opportunity cost of higher goods, is a phenomenon that baffled Augustine his entire life.[3] The best that might be said is that the second man is ignorant of the higher goods, but Augustine does not think we are capable of that degree of ignorance (Conf. 2.9). This man might just be longing for the feelings of virility and excitement of his now lost youth. But he is equating youth and excitement with the "shameful defilements" that Augustine was so tormented by in the Confessions. Youth, health and excitement are all good things, but not if they are wasted on sex. In Augustine's judgment, this man clearly and knowingly values the lower good of sex over the higher spiritual goods. In its most general form, this reordering of the moral hierarchy is an act of pride, an exaltation of our own value judgments in opposition to divine truth. This is Augustine's definition of moral wrong doing. Given Augustine's earliest writings on sex, desire, and sin, this second man has committed a much graver sin than the first. He has chosen to create a desire for sex when he must certainly know that he ought to desire chastity. A human being would only do something like this if he had decided, out of pride, that his value system was the correct one to follow.

3. Augustine's Mature Thoughts on Sex and Marriage

What is missing from this early condemnation of sex, and sexual desire, is any understanding of the genuine good of a faithful sexual marriage. Although celibate from his conversion (386ce), Augustine's more mature work shows a deeper understanding of the bonds of friendship and love that are formed in a sexual relationship. Augustine's understanding of sex and sexual desire is also more mature. He is aware of a mature man's inability to perform acts he was unable to refrain from in his youth. It is an older and wiser, but less virile Augustine, who wrote the passage above from the *City of God* (425ce).

It is customary to view the development of Augustine's thought as a response to heretics and other theological foes. The first two theological foes, the Manicheans and ascetics, argued that all sex was bad. The Manicheans believed that physical bodies were products of Darkness. Procreation trapped particles of Light in physical bodies preventing their return to their proper home. The ascetics, notably St. Jerome, argued that celibacy and virginity were the only sexual goods. For the ascetics, sex in a faithful marriage is not as bad a sin as fornication but it is still sin. Against these two Augustine argues that sex in marriage is not—in opposition to fornication—the lesser of two evils. Sex in marriage is—in opposition to celibacy—the the lesser of two goods. The third theological foe, the Pelagians, believed sexual desire was natural and sex in marriage was sinless. The Pelagians did not believe in original sin, and delighted in quoting Augustine's thoughts on the genuine good of a sexual marriage. Augustine responded to the Pelagians by expanding his view that a sexual marriage is a genuine good, but like all lesser goods it is fraught with difficulties. This would make Viagra a potentially useful tool, but a tool for gaining a good that is problematic in itself, and not the best thing a person could be striving for.

Augustine never came to accept sex, or sexual desire, as natural or unqualifiedly good. But he did come to believe that we can never gain voluntary control over our sexual desires. That degree of chastity, the voluntary elimination of all sexual lust, is not humanly possible in this life. Sexual desire always clashes with reason and will (C. Jul. 4.13.71; CG 14.16). For the mature Augustine sexual desire is as Peter Brown describes "a particularly resonant symptom of the frailty mankind inherited from Adam's first act of disobedience" (Brown, 1988, p. 416). It is our fallen nature and not our individual personal weakness that keeps people subjugated to sexual lust. Augustine didn't change his understanding of moral wrong doing. He did however come to argue that our unavoidable sexual lust can be channeled into a genuine lower good. Consequently an older more mature Augustine significantly softens the judgmental tone of his early condemnation of sexual desire.

4. Viagra and the Bonds of Friendship Formed in a Sexual Relationship

In the very first line of *On the Good of Marriage* Augustine tells us that "human nature is social" (OGM 1). We are created to form bonds with other human beings. The bonds of friendship between husband and wife and between parent and child are among the strongest and most significant human bonds. "When the spouses are old and unable to have intercourse" the marriage can continue to be a loving bond without sex but "marriage is not begun except through the union of bodies" (C. Jul. 5.16; OGM 9). This bond of friendship formed in a sexual marriage is the foundation for the three goods of marriage: children, fidelity, and sacrament. Each of these is a genuine good that grows only out of the bond of friendship formed in the expression of sexual love. None of these goods are part of a chaste life. The goods of marriage are different in kind, and can only be achieved in sexual marriage. When used properly to achieve and maintain these goods Viagra would be a useful and beneficial tool.

This bond, created and reinforced in a sexual relationship, is distinct from anything arising from lust. In our fallen state we experience sexual desire and the desire for the genuine love and companionship of marriage inextricably intertwined. But they are, in principle, separate (CG 14.10). There was sex in Eden before the fall, and there will be sex after the resurrection, when we return to our pre-fallen state: "It is the union of male and female sexually that forms the marriage and it is why male and female were created in Eden" (CG 14.22; 14.26).[4]

It is in our fallen state that this bond of a sexual marriage is fraught with difficulties. In a relatively recently discovered letter, dated around 421ce, a 67 year old Augustine draws a clear distinction between the lustful concupiscence of the flesh and the licit "concupiscence of conjugal purity, concupiscence of the legitimate engendering of children, or the concupiscence of the social bond by which each sex is tied to the other" (Ep. 6). The concupiscence of the flesh selfishly seeks only the pleasure of sex. The concupiscence of marriage seeks the goods of marriage: fidelity (conjugal purity), children, and friendship. Augustine's use of the word "concupiscence" is notable. Concupiscence is a desire for a lower good, a desire that can go wrong. So at the same time he is explaining that the desire for a faithful, sexual, married life is distinct from sexual lust, he is also warning us that the concupiscence of marriage is problematic.

Augustine's most cited passage on the bonds between spouses in a faithful sexual marriage affirms this good, but stresses moderation and the hope for eventual abstinence.

> In that Jesus came by invitation to a marriage, there is good ground to inquire for what reason marriage be a good. And this seems not to me to be merely on account of the begetting of children, but also on account of the natural friendship itself in a difference of sex. Otherwise it would not any longer be called marriage in the case of old persons, especially if either they had lost sons, or had given birth to none. But now in good, although aged, marriage, albeit there has withered away the glow of full age between male and female, yet there lives in full vigor the order of love between husband and wife: because, the better they are, the earlier they have begun by mutual consent to contain from sexual intercourse with each other: not that it should be matter of necessity afterwards not to have power to do what they would, but that it should be matter of praise to have been unwilling at the first, to do what they had power to do. If therefore there be kept good faith of honor, and of services mutually due from either sex, although the members of either be languishing and almost corpse-like, yet of souls duly joined together, the chastity continues, the purer by how much it is the more proved, the safer, by how much it is the calmer (OGM 3).

Augustine's Latin can be prosaic and hard to translate. This passage can appear almost dithering. He knows that he is expressing a view that many people will want to misunderstand, and seems unable to express a point fully before qualifying that point.[5] Nonetheless, a sexual marriage is good because of the natural friendship between two individuals of the opposite sex. Even when the couple is old and their members are corpse-like, there is still the bond of love that was formed and confirmed in their sexual relationship. This bond of love arises from moderation and mutual consideration of each other's needs (what is due from either sex). If the couple has been moderate, they have not necessarily been acting exclusively out of disordered lust (although lust plays a role). They will have a stronger bond of love and friendship than if they had been merely seeking to mutually satisfy their own lusts. They will also be better able to handle their coming impotence; their languishing and corpse-like members will not be the raging desirous disappointment described above. Mostly however they will be better prepared to seek the higher good of chastity.

Without ever losing sight of the fact that chastity is the higher good, Augustine confirms that sex can create, strengthen and reinforce the bond of love and friendship in a marriage. Viagra is not the preferred alternative, but it is a licit way of attaining this lower good. Chastity imposed by erectile dysfunction is not the mandatory end result of a marriage. In our old age we should hope and look forward to losing sexual desire. We should want to be free from lust, a freedom Augustine himself never enjoyed. But the desire for the bonds of friendship reinforced in a sexually active marriage is not sexual lust. In recognizing this as a good, even a lower good, Augustine is acknowledging that it can be properly pursued.

5. Viagra and the Three Goods of Marriage

The three goods of marriage, children, fidelity, and sacrament all grow out of the friendship and companionship of sexual marriage. Except for sacrament,[6] Viagra could help a couple attain these goods.

The connection between sex and children was well documented in Augustine's time. It is easy to see how Viagra might help a couple to conceive a child. It may be harder to fully understand why Viagra might help.

> Well, then, how significant is the fact that the eyes, and lips, and tongue, and hands, and feet, and the bending of back, and neck, and sides, are all placed within our power— to be applied to such operations as are suitable to them, when we have a body free from impediments and in a sound state of health; but when it must come to man's great function of the procreation of children the members which were expressly created for this purpose will not obey the direction of the will, but lust has to be waited for to set these members in motion, as if it had legal right over them, and sometimes it refuses to act when the mind wills (MC 1.7).

This is a common enough experience in men who are trying, without success, to conceive a child. It can be all but impossible to make yourself desire sex night after night after night. A man can desire to have a child. He may love his wife and desire her companionship. But in our fallen state it is just not possible to voluntarily make himself have sexual desire, and the "members will not obey the direction of the will."

This may be the one clear instance where Augustine would endorse use of Viagra. Taking Viagra is a voluntary act. If Viagra can inspire sexual desire and the ability to have sex then a man has regained some indirect control over his mind and body. Whether Viagra inspires his mind to lust or just his body to erection, he has acted voluntarily and subjugated these to a good purpose.

> Nevertheless conjugal intercourse is not in itself sin, when it is had with the intention of producing children; because the mind's good-will leads the ensuing bodily pleasure, instead of following its lead; and the human choice is not distracted by the yoke of sin pressing upon it, inasmuch as the blow of the sin is rightly brought back to the purposes of procreation (MC 1.13).

This works out even better for Augustine if Viagra causes physical ability but not sexual lust. Without sexual lust but merely the desire for companionship and children: "there is interposed a certain gravity of glowing pleasure, when in that wherein husband and wife cleave to one another, they have in mind that they be father and mother" (OGM 3). There is a distinct pleasure to purely procreative sex. This pleasure comes from the mind's good-will, not the genitals' stimulation.

This grave and glowing pleasure is quite different from the pleasure of lust inspired sex. Augustine has a great, flowering and expressive language to describe bodily pleasures.

> Lust not only takes possession of the whole body and outward members (…). The pleasure which results is the greatest of all bodily pleasures. (…) At the moment of time in which it is consummated, all mental activity is suspended (CG 14.16).

Augustine can write, from vivid memory, of the mind numbing pleasure offered by the momentary satisfaction of sexual lust. The best he can offer about the pleasure of the higher good is "grave and glowing." But it is a higher pleasure nonetheless. The experiential difference is maybe this. When one remembers lustful sexual ecstasy, the memory is a dim reflection of past momentary pleasure. On the other hand one does not merely remember the higher pleasures; to call them to mind is to experience them again. The higher pleasures have a lasting permanence that is perhaps best described as "grave and glowing."

Annie Potts argues that Viagra allows the body to be reprogrammed, removing sexual desire as a necessary element in producing an erection (Potts, 2004, p. 227). She views this negatively as the removal of the authenticity of the sexual experience. Augustine would likely have just the opposite assessment. Viagra may allow a man to experience the higher pleasure purely, unmixed with lust. By producing the erection through the voluntary use of pharmaceuticals, a man can seek the goods of marriage, in this case children and companionship, but also pleasure, without lust. Augustine thought it was impossible in our fallen state to even imagine what it would be like to experience the goods of marriage, including sexual pleasure, without lust (CG 14.23-24). If Viagra creates the physical ability, without inspiring lust, then the result would seem to be close to the sexual experience of the first humans in Paradise. Potts perhaps shares the opinion of the twelfth-century theologian William of Champeaux, who comments that sex in Paradise was no more pleasurable than "putting your finger in your mouth" (Champeaux, 1959, p. 254). But this is only because they don't understand the higher pleasure.

The second good of marriage, fidelity, is not merely marital fidelity as it is currently understood—not having sex with other people. Fidelity for Augustine is a mutual obligation to provide your spouse with a licit and permissible outlet for sexual energies (OGM 6; MC 2.53). It is this mutual commitment between two individuals that makes even lustful sex pardonable in marriage (OGM 6). Late in his life Augustine still carried some of the baggage of his earlier views. He still thought that people get married because they are not strong enough to be celibate. His more mature view is that a weak couple can create a genuine good by supporting each other in their mutual weakness, and channeling their lust into a lawful marriage that is open to the possibility of children. He does not view this sexual obligation as transactional—as one spouse performing a service and getting some benefit in return. Fidelity is a mutual pact to assist each other, so that neither spouse is driven by lust to an act that might damn their soul. Augustine writes as if the couple is helping each other with a particularly distasteful task.

Because the good attained by fidelity is a licit and less sinful release of lust, erectile dysfunction can be especially disruptive to marital fidelity. There are three possible scenarios: both spouses are driven by lust to desire sex, but the man has erectile dysfunction; second, the woman has no desire for sex, the man has erectile dysfunction but takes Viagra; third, the woman is driven by lust to desire sex but the man has either low libido or erectile dysfunction.

In the first case there is a clear motive to use Viagra. For this couple, Viagra is just a useful tool in their mutual attempt to support each other's sexual weakness. The fact that they are giving in to lust is pardonable in a faithful marriage. Viagra here may prevent the man from experiencing the raging desirous shame described above. It may prevent the woman from committing adultery. This couple is motivated by carnal or sexual concupiscence. They have not practiced the moderation Augustine wrote of above, but their use of Viagra is good insofar as their fidelity is a mutual pact of assistance. It is a genuine good because they are helping each other to maintain lawful discipline and proper order in their sexual lusts. This couple's use of Viagra is not as morally good as the couple described above who are motivated by concupiscence of marriage and use Viagra to reinforce the bonds of marital friendship.

Case two and three are significantly different from the first. Augustine is quite clear and explicit that each spouse has a sexual obligation whether he or she has any sexual desire or not. In a letter Augustine chastises an otherwise unknown woman, Ecdicia, who had chosen to live chastely after many years of marriage. Augustine reaffirms that as a couple ages, if they mutually agree, their fidelity can become mutual support in the attempt to achieve the higher good of chastity. However, Ecdicia's husband did not agree to live chastely. Augustine condemns her for driving the man to fornication and adultery (Ep. 262). Most of these cases seem to involve women who want to be chaste and men who do not. Even if it is just hypothetical, Augustine is quick to point out that either the male or female spouse may be required to "yield what is due, observing in all things a loving and religious concord" (OGM 15). He tells Ecdicia that had her husband been the one seeking chastity, "he would have been obliged to render you the debt, and God would have given him credit for continence if he had not refused you marital intercourse, out of consideration for your weakness not his own, in order to prevent you from falling into the damnable sin of adultery" (Ep. 262). This mutual obligation would seem to make the duty in the second and third cases clear. Either spouse is obligated to provide sexual service.

In the second case, absent the man's taking Viagra, his wife would not have to consent to perform her duty. For all the reasons discussed earlier the man should not take Viagra. With erectile dysfunction and or low libido he is unlikely to commit adultery. It is possible that a man might need Viagra to desire and have sex with his wife, but not with another woman. Thus his taking Viagra would in fact be a preferable alternative. But, unlike the later scholastics and contemporary analytic philosophers, Augustine is generally unmoved by this kind of rationalizing "just so" story. In this second case the man is seeking the release of sexual lust not the goods of marital friendship. Nonetheless, once the man has taken Viagra it would be the wife's duty to have sex with him.

In the third case the woman is driven by lust to desire sex but the man has either low libido or erectile dysfunction. In one of his more crass observations, Augustine notes that a disinterested woman has a fairly easy time participating physically in sex (OGM 10). She can just lie there and think of Carthage. Just lying there is exactly the problem with a disinterested man. This man would be obligated to use Viagra in order to fulfill his duties. He had agreed when they got married to assist his wife in her sexual weakness. So Viagra may continue the good of fidelity. But this man's dutiful sex will not give him the grave and glowing pleasure of pursuing sex out of pure desire for the good of marital friendship and children.

On this point Augustine just seems to just misunderstand human nature. This mutual obligation to be used as a receptacle for your partner's lust can seriously undermine the bonds of friendship in a marriage. Anecdotally both women and men report that the possibility of Viagra use makes this problem worse (Loe, 2004, p. 108ff; Croissant, 2006; Potts, 2003). There is an expectation on the part of the dutiful partner that, with old age, there will be less demand for sex. For women content with their own lower sex drive, the possibility of their husband's taking Viagra is not something they look forward to. For men uninterested in sex, the need to use Viagra can exacerbate the perceived sense of inadequacy. It is harder to claim that low male libido is natural when it can be medicalized as erectile dysfunction, and "cured" with a pill. This is a point of human sexuality that Augustine just doesn't seem to understand. There is a sense in which a married couple has made a commitment to support each other in their weaknesses. But where this support involves the most intimate of human acts, it simply cannot be continually demanded without an erosion of the bonds of love and friendship. Pharmaceutical enhancement of sexual desire and performance can only raise the level of difficulty in rendering this mutual support.

Viagra could be a useful and beneficial tool, but one that must be used wisely. Viagra has the possibility of enhancing the companionship that grows in the sexual bond of marriage, but it also has the possibility of destroying that bond. Viagra can add to the difficulty a couple has in moderately and appropriately pursuing a lower good. The safest option it still abstinence. "Many indeed with more ease practice abstinence, so as not to use, than practice temperance, so as to use well" (OGM 25). Viagra makes moderation harder.

What of the couple that uses Viagra out of the desire to reinforce the genuine bonds of friendship in a sexual marriage? How could the concupiscence of marriage go wrong? The defining trait of a lower good is that it can be sought excessively and to one's harm. This was true of the first man, Adam, who, "could not bear to be severed from his only companion, even though this involved a partnership in sin. He was not on this account less culpable, but sinned with his eyes open" (CG 14.11). Adam's desire was uncorrupted by lust. He experienced the pure desire for marital companionship. Because marital friendship is a lower good it is possible to love one's spouse too much (cf. Clark, 1986). Adam placed a value on marital friendship well beyond its true worth. He went wrong in desiring Eve's companionship too much. The real danger for Augustine would come when individuals wrongly judge the goods of marriage to be superior to goods attained in the love and worship of God. The goods of a sexual marriage can be enjoyed, "provided however it be not so in excess as to hinder what ought to be set aside as seasons of prayer" (OGM 11). Adam knowingly turned aside from God because he valued Eve's friendship and companionship. Until he sinned, Adam did not even experience lust. In our fallen state sex is the greatest physical pleasure we can experience. So far removed from God, we are much more likely to go wrong. Even those people who experience this concupiscence for marital friendship experience it thoroughly intermixed with sexual lust and sexual pleasure. If Viagra allows more and better sex it artificially enhances the physical pleasure without necessarily enhancing the other bonds of friendship. This makes Viagra a dangerous, but effective, tool for achieving a lower good. One to be used with great caution, but probably better avoided.

The most Augustinian fact in the current Viagra research is that only a small percentage of men ever get prescriptions for Viagra. Of these, 60% do not renew the prescription (Marshall, 2006, p. 352). Augustine's final word on Viagra would likely be the same as his final word on sex itself. "Such is the weakness of the flesh, such is the irksome nature of this life, that everything, however wonderful ends in boredom" (Sermon 243, Miles, 2005).

Notes

1. Hunter 1994 and Meileander 2001 discuss the extensive literature on Augustine's pessimistic views of sex. Both take a more optimistic view. Pagels (1988 chap. 5) argues that Augustine's description of the effects of the sexual nature of orig-

inal sin and the resulting loss of human freedom served to justify the coercive power of the imperial church. Burke (1990) is one recent polemical attempt to bring Augustine into the conversation on current sexual morality. Burke cites extensively the use of Augustine by the Congregation for the Doctrine of the Faith (nee The inquisition).

2. I am not qualified to assess the real effects of Viagra. There are questions about whether Viagra can produce sexual desire by creating an erection, or whether Viagra simply creates an erection. It may be that any increase in desire is the placebo effect arising from the removal of anxiety. What is important for Augustine is that men seek Viagra thinking that it will either boost their libido, give them erections, or both. (cf. Boisaubin and McCullough 2004; Marshall 2006)
3. See Confessions Book 2 where Augustine describes the worst sin he ever committed in his life as the petty theft of some pears. It was truly wrong because he stole only because he knew theft was a sin. D.C. Shindler (2005) has an excellent recent discussion of Augustine's thoughts on why and how we make such foolish and immoral choices.
4. Augustine must acknowledge that Mary and Joseph were properly married although they (as some Catholics claim) never had sex. But that degree of perfection is supererogatory (MC 1.12).
5. Meilaender (2001), for example, takes this passage as an endorsement of contraception. Augustine is always and explicitly clear in asserting that the couple need not intend to have children but must be open to the possibility of children (MC 1.9; 1.16). This is the root of the Catholic policy that rules out active contraception but allows the rhythm method.
6. Sacrament is the commitment to live as a Christian married couple. It differentiates Christians from other sects that may have advocated a similar sexual lifestyle but not out of love of Christ.

Five

VIAGRA AND THE UTOPIA OF IMMORTALITY

Robert Redeker

1. Introduction

In order to understand the philosophical scope of Viagra we have to put it into the context of a collective fantasy of a new body and of a new idea of the human being. Viagra is not an isolated phenomenon. Nor is it merely a medicine healing a disease. More than a medicine, it represents an anthropological rupture. Historically speaking, most drugs have remained anthropologically continuous, that is, they did not radically transform the perception of the human body. Viagra on the other hand, appears like a bridge leading from an older concept of the human to a newer, entirely different one. Viagra inaugurates the existence of a new man and in that sense, it is part and parcel of a utopia which, contrary to those of past centuries that were always held together by explicit theories, has no conceptual center that can be analyzed or criticized.

What exactly is this new body? What is this new man? What are the features of the Viagra-based utopia? The body imagined by Viagra is not just any body. It is not the body that people have had for thousands of years. It is not the body that we tend to call a "natural body" (which is, by the way, an imprecise expression because the body has always been a mixture of nature and culture). The old body was the recipient of diseases, submitted to care and to medical treatment. The old body was always thought of within a series of relationships often adopting the form of oppositions: body vs. spirit, body vs. soul, body vs. ancestors; it was the body seen in relationship with time and death. It was conceived of as frail and weak and its ultimate destiny was obsoleteness. The body in the era of Viagra conceives itself as invincible. This body no longer needs anything that is opposed to itself nor does it need anything that is made of another ontological fabric in order to preserve its existence.

In the history of humanity, the Viagra body is a complete novelty. Its outlines have been visible in pornographic cinema, in advertisements, and in sport. The Viagra body is not the Platonic body inhabited by a soul, nor is it the body whose soul is conceived as an Aristotelian form. It is not the "corps propre" upon which Maine de Biran meditates, nor is it Descartes' body as a machine. Our present body is an appliance (*corps-appareil*).

Viagra does not create the machine-man of La Mettrie, but an entity which, so far, no philosopher has ever referred to: the appliance-man. The mechanic model of the body—used by Descartes and later by La Mettrie—

would lead to Newtonian physics. The model of the appliance, on the other hand, leads straight towards a string of other sciences such as chemistry, electronics, quantum physics, and cybernetics. Viagra does not transform the human into Vaucanson's automaton working, under Cartesian influence, with pulleys and belts. Viagra transforms the human being into an engine determined by the circulation of energy. This is the appliance-man. The difference between a machine and an appliance is like that between a clock relying only on its mechanics having to be wound up every day and a clock functioning with batteries.

Like the machine-man, the appliance-man has no free will. With Viagra, liberty has disappeared because, from the beginning, it is clear that the parts needed for the sexual act will "function." Liberty presupposes incertitude. Therefore, Viagra negates the will as much as liberty within the realm of sexuality.

The new body without soul is also a body without self: it is an unspirited (*désanimé*) and de-egotized (*déségoïsé*) body. In the case of the Viagra-body, it has become impossible to separate soul/self or psyche/ego from body because this body has *absorbed* both the soul and the self. This is the reason why I name it "egobody."[1]

What is or what was the self if not the place of identity troubles? Søren Kierkegaard's nervous dialogue between the self and the Gospels illustrates the relationship between the 'I' and a permanent "trembling." According to the philosopher from Copenhagen, "the self cannot of itself attain and remain in equilibrium and rest by itself" (Kierkegaard, 2008, p. 10). Unamuno's thesis of faith as agony from *The Agony of Christ* is very relevant here. In other words, the self is agony, battle and doubt. Viagra suppresses this constitutive battle of the self and by doing so, it depsychologizes and de-egotizes sexuality. More precisely: since sexuality, like any activity of the self, implies incertitude and is defined through the above battle, Viagra desexualizes sexuality. Sexuality visited by Viagra is identifiable with what is exhibited in pornographic cinema: it is everything but sexuality (sexuality is actually absent also from that type of cinema).

2. Sexuality and Space

Sexuality, when submitted to incertitude, was rather like Descartes' pineal gland. It was a place where body and soul could meet and face each other. Michel Foucault's analysis or the pastorals of the Counter-Reformation permits the attentive reader to get an idea of how much Christian Europe has been aware of this encounter (Foucault, 1976, pp. 26-30). In reality, for the Catholic tradition since Saint Paul, the crossroad called sexuality was the place where the soul could be lead into perdition. It is here, in sexuality, that the soul could lose itself.

Today the place of sexuality is very different from the Cartesian pineal gland. The pineal gland would occupy a distinct place in the brain where it could be localized and removed with the scalpel. The pineal gland existed within an extension, which is not the case with sexuality because it can be neither removed nor grafted. Only death—once defined by the Platonic tradition as the separation of the soul from the body—can put a radical end to sexual activities.

Even though it is possible to surgically or chemically suppress the back-ups of sexuality, once it is understood as a mere libido or a vital energy, it becomes impossible to suppress it ontologically. Today, sexuality is no longer present in the mode of being that Descartes, following the scholastics, had called "extension." For Descartes, the pineal gland structures body and soul. Freud offers a different message to the modern world, and his message was meant as a sublime suggestion to resist modern materialism: the above structuring process would take place in sexuality. However, this place called sexuality is a non-place. It is the sexual instinct, it is the libido, and thus energy rather than an organ. Contrary to Descartes' pineal gland where body and soul meet, Freud's sexuality (which is a function or, when rendered in the form of the libido, an energy), is a non-topical place. Freud's discovery can be summarized as such: On the one hand, sexuality can be localized; on the other hand, when seen as libido, it cannot be localized. It is not absurd to suppose that Freud attempted—perhaps unwillingly—to protect the soul, an entity threatened by the progress of positivist and neurological psychology.

How can the soul be saved during the age of science? How can a notion be saved whose philosophical origin goes back to Plato before undergoing a thousand transformations at the hands of Aristotle, Saint Augustine, Descartes, Malebranche, and Spinoza? A notion, which has been greatly transformed by psychoanalysis, a science that will always remain materialistic or even deterministic though never biologistic. Popper was not mistaken: psychoanalysis invents a discourse on the soul disguised by the habits of science, thus passing as scientific. By inventing psychoanalysis, Freud makes the scientific analysis of the soul possible by using strange methods. Through the libido he energizes sexuality, that is, he dis-places sexuality. Before Freud, such dis-placements had been attacked by the clergy. According to St. Augustine, the libido is the path where the soul gets lost. Freud retrieves the term "libido," inverts its direction, and uses it to save the soul.

3. The Mental

What is this new man? It is a being whose soul, self, and body have been fused in order to engender a new entity. Besides the new body, there is another function that appears upon the ruins of the soul and the self: the mental. The new man no longer has a soul or a self, but he has a psyche. The mental occupies the place of the new man's "psychism." For the new man, the mental is the analogue of what used to be the soul and the self for earlier forms of humanity. According to Max Stirner, the "Man and the I are synonymous" (Avron, 1973, p. 156). Today it is better to talk of the identity of the self (ego) and the new body which negates the self. The new body is the grave of the self, just like for Plato (in the *Phaedo*) the body is the grave of the soul. The mental is not more than the result of this negation of the self within the new body. The existence of the mental represents two movements at the same time. It represents the reduction of the psychological function to muscle power and the reduction of the self and of the soul to a muscle. Sometimes this mental is on the winning side, sometimes it is on the losing side. Through the mental we can view the activities of psychological life (the life of the psyche) as if it were a sport. It goes without saying that Viagra-assisted sexuality is most suitable for an age where the psyche has become a muscle. As a matter of fact, neither the self nor the soul can be used for the purposes of Viagra.

4. Cosmos and Cosmetics

The masculine Viagra finds a parallel in women's modified approach towards cosmetics. Cosmetics have been wrenched from its origin, which is the emulations of the cosmos' universal beauty. Traditionally, cosmetics intended, through its artifices, to highlight feminine beauty as the microcosmos of cosmic beauty. In other words, cosmetics exalted both beauty and the cosmos. Now the main task of cosmetics has become to repair. Cosmetics is no longer satisfied with the *masking* of time and death, but it provides the illusion that it can *repair* those effects that death, wrinkles, the dryness of cells, etc. have left on the body. It is no longer the obsession with beauty that legitimizes its existence, but the obsession with death. In this sense, the current use of cosmetics comes close to embalming and thanatopraxis even though those who are "embalmed" are still alive. The new cosmetics are no longer related to beauty, but to death as it attempts to mask the advancement of death with the help of anti-aging products and regenerative strategies. The principle idea is no longer to put the woman in relationship with the harmony of the cosmos but—quite to the contrary—to dissimulate as much as possible the work of nature, that is, to disharmonize the relationship between the female body and nature. Therefore both the masculine Viagra and feminine cosmetics are of the same order; they go hand-in-hand and function, in spite of their thanatopractical aspect, within a unique dream of immortality. Denying time and death, they aspire to eternal life.

We understand that Viagra articulates nothing less than a new utopia. In the past, utopias used to be explicit theories, clearly conceptualized, offering the detailed outline of an ideal existence, and attempting to elaborate an ideal type of society. This is not the case with the utopia of Viagra. In spite of this, there is something that Viagra and the old utopia have in common. Campanella's utopia required that love become automatized and mechanized, just as with Viagra. His utopia required that sex be carried out at certain hours that would be fixed by the authorities beforehand. This aspect of utopian thought anticipates a major trait of Viagra in political philosophy though it also resembles pornographic cinema implying the disconnection of sexuality from liberty, that is, the desexualization of sexuality.

Our present utopia of Viagra is not *explicit* like Campanella's, but *implicit*, meandering between different human practices. Far from materializing these practices through governmental orders, the present utopia remains in the realm of the unspoken. The reason is certainly that the Viagra utopia is more of a wish than a program. What I mean is the utopia of immortality. We have to insist on the originality of contemporary immortalism because it neither accomplishes nor continues religious thought, but revokes it. The majority of religious movements offer some sort of immortality after having passed the threshold of death, which acquires, in turn, the status of an initiation. The immortalist utopia that permeates the age of Viagra, on the other hand, excludes the experience of death. Instead it dreams of an immortality ante-mortem, an immortality that does not need to go through the needle's eye of death. This utopia scorns the paradox represented by an immortality extant within extension, an immortality staged within entropic space. As a consequence, the immortality of Viagra's utopia is inherent and not transcendental, as is the one described by Saint Augustine in *The City of God.* The immortality of Viagra is obtained not through a spiritual effort, but through industriousness.

5. Conclusion

From an anthropological point of view, 1988, the year of the discovery of Viagra, is extremely important because it announces the arrival of a new type of man to which all of us will have to assimilate. This man is equipped with a new (fantasmatically infallible) body and with a mental capacity that serves as a substitute for the soul and the self. This product will manage to reconfigure sexuality in its totality. Sexuality, which was once able to draw the demarcation line between humans and animals, is now desexualized and introduced into the realm of pornographic cinema. To use Viagra is to enter the community or the communion (as if the taking of the blue pill were a parody of the holy sacrament) of a new type of human being.

Translated from the French by TBB.

Note

1. *Egobody* is also the title of Robert Redeker's newest book (Paris: Fayard, 2010).

Six

ENHANCING DESIRE PHILOSOPHICALLY: FEMINISM, VIAGRA, AND THE BIOPOLITICS OF THE FUTURE

Connie C. Price

1. Introduction

Prior to the invention of Viagra, the medical community had reached a consensus that erectile dysfunction is a physiological problem rather than, as had been assumed for many years, a psychological one.[1] The decision shows an unfortunate habit in medical and bioethical discourse, namely the insistence that one side of a postulated dichotomy must be chosen, as the correct basis for future research. The gender dichotomy is false; and sex, with all its problems, is an area where the line between physiology and psychology is especially blurred. Further, when sex and desire are considered from a feminist perspective, it becomes evident that sex, including attitudes, imaging, and behaviors regarding the sexual organs, is a social phenomenon, a political one, and indeed, an ontological one. All three of these areas merit attention, to develop better understanding of the overwhelming market success of the blue pill and its cousins. Nor must the physiological and psychological concerns be ignored. For example, perhaps scholars of sexuality need to reexamine the meaning of Freud's concept of the death wish. He may have been arguing that life has disappeared from human institutions, and that is why society does not seem to be able to create any justice. Thus, today's crises of the schools, of food and nutrition, and yes, of sexual practices, are intertwined. The challenge to revitalize society is where the political side comes into controversies about sex and desire and the band-aid remedy, Viagra. This is a more holistic politics than that of the gender wars, which have comprised perhaps by necessity the basis of feminist philosophy, up until the present day. There are even evolutionary implications in feminist *prise de parole*. Developing a discourse which is sexual, and yet is not obsessed materialistically upon measurements and tumescence, involves overcoming secrecy and shame. Such moral transformations in speech and emotional power would contribute to phenotypical change, as conceptualized by Bergson, Nietzsche, Whitehead, Bateson, and Deleuze.

To begin a reflection on the significance of Viagra for feminist philosophy, one can consider a hypothetical example, a conventional and typical case. A couple have had trouble with their relationship, and are considering a breakup. In therapy sessions they have articulated clearly for the first time that their only issue is their sex life. The future of their marriage, then, turns 'round a "single issue," but it seems for this couple to be an overwhelming and irresolvable issue. Furthermore, neither partner wants to continue a relationship where sex is disappointing or nonexistent. Although the example may be a clichéd opener for a self-help or pop psychology publication, a philosophical direction can also be taken from its context. Such a philosophy is rooted in a combination of feminist, political, and ethical concerns. These theoretical approaches, and in particular the justification for merging them as a coherent philosophy, are based in the thought of Henri Bergson, the American pragmatists including Susanne Langer, continental feminism, and the new movements (1960's-2010's) in Bergsonian, Nietzschean, and Freudian thought. This robust school was for some time known as contemporary continental thought, postmodernism, post-structuralism, neo-vitalism, and other titles, but is now usually called biopolitics. Originating in the mid-nineteenth century, the ideas of the movement have to do with producing radical values, one of the most outrageous of which was the view that women ought to be assigned to the realm of reality. Although it is granted that sexism has continued to be evident in many authors in this area of philosophy, the very fact of placing female existence in the world as an entity other than breeder, an ethical entity whose feelings and thoughts are part of the daily life of speech, values, and events, is a feminist rupture in thought and it had no precedent before Kierkegaard and Marx.

Out of this philosophical base emerges an approach that in contrast may seem simplistic for resolving the sexual problems of the frustrated couple introduced above: failure to consider feelings has led the couple into a disastrous situation. If the two were to come to terms with their emotions, they might be able to decide their future course more confidently. A bit nostalgically, one can ask "What if?" and consider the possibility that they may have encountered one another from the time of their first meeting or first attraction, not in terms of the man's anatomical comportment, but of their feelings for each other. Their chances are not good, from this point forward, for beginning a life of feelings together. Long-term work with a humanistic style of psychotherapy such as the phenomenological or family systems approaches, might help them (Kerr, 1988). Such an endeavor would require a boot camp of sorts, a complete immersion in treatment, possibly for years on end. This would be the only way yet known to learn the habits of emotive relationship while at the same time unlearning those of an anatomical and material relationship. This is not to say that the couple must learn to absent themselves from sex and one another's bodies and communicate in shrink speak. To the contrary, the goal in psychiatric boot camp, marital feelings 101, would be to become embodied sexual partners, free from certain behaviors they have come to associate with a normal relationship, including a tendency to measure anatomical parts as an indication of one's or one another's actual desire and passion, or to compare one's partner's appearance with that of film stars and models, or to spend one's cash on instruments of bondage, such as bikini waxes, painted toenails, and high heeled shoes. Dating and romances are always already built from emotional discourses that can become an excellent beginning for a sexual lifetime together, a philosophical turning that needs to come to the surface of the cultural understanding of courtship. Such sexual talking[2] must continue throughout a marriage, at the same degree of cognitive richness that is taken on when first attraction occurs. Over time, a couple become aware that new feelings have emerged in their partnering. They learn to regard themselves as inventors of new emotions and even new levels of feeling. The sexual being of their private dialogues has to be attended and consciously developed rather than being edited out of their daily habits and replaced by appliances and cruise packages. If a couple receive guidance and continue their efforts in "sex feeling speak" through the years, it is not certain that they will live happily ever after together, but their support for one another's dignity is likely to set a moral example for others, and if parting becomes necessary, they are better prepared to cherish and befriend one another.

2. Biopolitics and Viagra: Affective Justice as the Evolution of the Future

The importance of politics—that is, of building and nurturing institutions that constitute a free life-world—is ignored at great peril in controversies about sex and desire, including responses to the current band-aid remedy, Viagra. Sexual problems are political problems. Before the era of feminism, this statement could refer only to the dour systems of misogyny. Today, perceiving sex as a topic requiring political attention means that sexual issues are questions related to the neo-vitalistic concept of will to power with emphasis on the course of evolution of the future, developed by Nietzsche's, Bergson's, and related philosophies. Feminists must engage these issues, and must change the language and the life of desire to a vast degree. The feminist project of the future will be the creation of affective justice (Price, 2006; Protevi, 2009). The convenient association, one that seems to be presupposed as authentic in typical discussions about sex, must be broken. That association is between on the one hand, sexual slavery and repression and on the other, women's existence, rights, and creations of destiny. Feminism smashes this associative idol, creating instead a discourse of unfettered deepening of inwardness. For this reason, feminism comprises evolutionary growth for humanity, an event which Kierkegaard, Nietzsche, Bergson, and the contemporary thinkers in the biopolitical tradition, have considered necessary if ethics were ever to begin. The gender wars, and thus the globally pervasive cultural habit of reducing women's desire to a codependent means of survival, must come to an end, in feminist evolution. The transformative events that are involved in a more mature and evolutionary perspective on sexual rejuvenation have the potential for returning the world to its originative ways of love and desire, a cultural shock more powerful than Viagra has brought on and also more lasting in its affirmation of sexual health. "Originative" in this context means, not a utopian projection of the emotive past, recalled wistfully, but rather, the creative ability to begin anew to define and experience love. Speaking desire has potential for helping people understand sexual problems. In healthcare settings, solutions may emerge that are not as invasive as Viagra is. People begin to create bonds as sexual beings whose shared feelings are their relationship's priorities. The fact that there are sexual problems to resolve becomes an affirmation of a relationship, not its destroyer. It is time to tell some new myths in a new speech. Better yet, it is time to outgrow the narrative sense of consciousness. Stories may and must there always be, but let them be told with cultural honesty. Stories are an art, and for that reason only, are they necessary. In the tales of the future, let feelings and justice be one, so that actual sexual disorders are those that fall short of commensurate feelings rather than comprising failures to perform in the graphic anatomical compulsions which Homo sapiens has until now reserved as its only love story. Such new myths must take heart in the concerns, habits, relationships, emotions, and conversations of ordinary people.

Discourses which generate from a shared commitment to affective justice, be the discourses academic, governmental, or communitarian, would sustain more interesting and promising politics than the gender wars have done. War by definition decimates women's desires, their ways of living and expression, their safety, and their leadership. Destruction of the feminine is the purpose of war, not merely one of war's collateral damages. Feminism has to transform its own discourse and by implication all discourses. This is precisely the sort of change which is inhibited by masculinism and misogyny, for untold reasons and agendas. In the gender wars, ideas fail in the Platonic eros of being gadflies, compelling human encounters through ecstasy and language instead of violence. When speaking desire becomes a norm in the vernacular, politics can change sexual lives for the better, and in a reciprocal way, folk can for the first time in history become both political and ethical. Evolutionary potential exists in the creation of a discourse that is sexual, and yet is not inscribed as a fetish. It is fortunate that geneticists, or more correctly their hagiographers in the human sciences and the media, have not yet grabbed onto the notion that sexual dysfunctions may be genetic in origin. Ironically it may have been Viagra, despite its negative impact on sexual politics, that has had the important affirmative value of offsetting, up to the present at least, genetic interventions of the sort that are now attempted for many other ailments. In today's fractious medical world, once the genetic origins of a disease or defect are preyed upon for research grants, prizes, media attention, and teaching points, all bets are off for continuing to interrogate issues such as the meaning of health and illness, or the spiritual and social impact of proposed treatments, among the disciplines in the liberal arts: philosophy, ethics, clinical psychology, history, linguistics. Feminists need to seize this precious gap time! For example, regarding the crucial evolutionary significance of sexual functions and dysfunctions, once the very insight that a relation exists between evolution and a society's chosen concepts of sexual functions (a philosophical breakthrough which Kierkegaard, Nietzsche, Marx, Freud, and Bergson were calling for), were to be appropriated by the geneticists, and especially their groupies, e.g. Dawkins, Dennett, etc., still another discursive obstacle would exist against the telling of desire and feelings. Viagra can be understood as having helped demolish the barrier that the concept of genetic origins of diseases inevitably poses against human expression about health and illness. Unfortunately, offsetting the popular genes speak from treatments for male sexual dysfunction has occurred through the dubious route of contributing to the illusion that sexual desire is a free element of consciousness suitable for oversimplified medical interventions. The new blue pill's enhancement of the ability to act more freely within the given logistics of sexual desire and intercourse diminishes even further the least free aspect of women's repressed lives, and enables the freest, perhaps the only free, aspect of men's repressed lives. Even as Viagra was designed for easier fulfillment of both sexes' one alleged desire, so must it be recalled that historically it remains the case that among the accumulated unconscious sexual significations of the human psyche, only men's desires and not women's are free. At least is this the case, according to the social norms that are longstanding and deeply ingrained from narratives told by the powerful throughout the ages, e.g. from the modernists' contracted and mechanistic ideologies; from the positivistic, sociobiological center of mythmaking, namely the academic and industrial machine known as the biosciences; and from the canonically spiritual locus for the production of myths, the churches. The controlling power of the belief systems now issuing from these various discursive centers goes unquestioned by any agency of resistance except for the feminist biopolitical movement. For example, no efforts by clergy or laity, even in the most liberal denominations, have yet been offered, to give a hermeneutical reading of the passage in the Bible, in Genesis, where, upon Adam and Eve's expulsion from The Garden, women are condemned to desire and crave their husbands for all of their (the women's) days. As this has played out in civilization, if she is single, a woman's desires are by implication distorted, frustrated, and untrustworthy. Such women are the witches of the woods, the stand-up comics, the female philosophers. With the massive acceptance of Viagra, the culture revives this religious decree, which may appear superficially to assimilate Nietzsche's philosophy, but does not include the crucial evolutionary sense that Nietzsche intended. Instead, this false "return" would be a rerun, a repetition, mechanistic and based on the Newtonian spatiotemporal physics: at last, a pill restores men's natural and universal behavioral choices! Since the birth control pill and the sexual revolution of the 1960's, and now with Viagra to keep the illusions intact for awhile longer, women also now have the wondrous liberty to respond to the graphics, the cartoon reality, of their male partners' genitals! Beginning in 1960, straight women's sexual practice follows one simple and easy rule: whatever he says, she will do. His body, graphically reconfigured by medical research now with Viagra, can be relied upon to express his one-dimensional expectations. As for her, she has even less recourse than before, to negotiate sexual terms with him; nor does she seem to be aware of such discursive options. Never mind that women's desires may not be of a graphic nature at all, to say nothing of being genital and related to size or to degrees of tumescence and hardness. Her spoken desires are not at issue in the marketing and consumption of drugs for phallic enhancement! According to the current bioscientific urmyth, women cannot expect to express in words or images their actual erotic desires any more readily than was possible before the advent of Viagra, because all sexual expectations are presumed to center and now to recenter on male genitals.

An ethical consideration of issues surrounding Viagra demonstrates the conservatism of bioethics as it has been pursued for some forty years. Engaging the ethics of Viagra requires bioethics to pay attention to radical feminist politics. Viagra tends to reinforce a view of sex and of heterosexual relationships as instituted in the human race for the purpose of gratifying men's needs while ignoring, trivializing, and mocking those of women. There seems to be little if anything about Viagra that serves to counteract the violence and abuse of women that have been part of the traditions in courtship and marriage throughout the ages. Nor do the enduring practices of prostituting women's sexual lives and considering pornography as the best way to depict images of the female body seem to be undermined by the advent of Viagra. The image of male sexuality as a process of trafficking in women's emotions is universal among cultures, and no reflection or restraint on this abuse is taken by the pharmaceutical industry. Heterosexuality has regressed into a numbers game, placing the stakes on measurements and a material view of itself. Viagra has encouraged this false return, retrospectively: an unheeded phallocentric backlash regarding desire was never silent in literature, architecture, the formation of totalitarian regimes, or the rise of positivistic science and medicine, earlier on, back as far as Kierkegaard's feminist manifesto (Kierkegaard, 1983). It stands to reason that male-oriented life and culture would have been threatened by philosophical and theological initiatives encouraging women's prise de parole, actualizing for the first time in history a feminist meaning of desire. Feminist desire is destined unlike phallic desire to be more in keeping with sex as an evaluative dynamic of life in ways comparable to the significance of such phenomena as thinking, creating, and feeling (Merleau-Ponty, 1962). What if there were a pill for the major social crises, such as the pandemics of both hunger and obesity, the conditions of the schools, and even infrastructural crises such as oil spills, smog, and the failing roads and bridges? Might the citizenry buy these capsules and ingest them, as prescribed for optimum results?

3. Affective Justice Radicalizes the Political Topos

In an updated Freudian sense, massive refusal and self-deception about sex are evident. People don't want to accept the fact that sex and intercourse are political, even apart from and in a more persuasively significant way than is acknowledged by the dichotomous set-up of women known as the gender wars. It is possible after all for discourses about sex to be sociopolitical on a par with food and education. Sex can become one of the elements of building democracy. Issues about food and education are no more successfully articulated today than sexual desire is. To be resolved, all three issues and many others including healthcare, street and domestic violence, drugs, and border conflicts, require mutual commitment to developing a better society. These perplexing issues are of course interrelated. Compartmentalizing them is itself an example of technocapital's production of a fragmented psyche, an effort which cognitive science supports. It is necessary to discern and articulate relations among social issues. Perhaps it would be well to forge new connections as part of the discussions, and indeed the solutions. The compulsion to be secretive and hushed about "that one thing" does much social harm. Inevitable reactions to this brittle secretiveness, reactions which themselves often receive public recognition as social problems, include creating a prohibition-style pornographic industry and promoting rape as the model of sex and as the one acceptable war crime. After all, who's kidding who? Children's knowledge and their talk are immersed in porn today. Adults like to pretend otherwise and keep it a secret that the secret is out. However, harms that are even more devastating than turning parenthood into the lucrative production of future markets in porn, rape, and prostitution, may come from the rampant shame and secrecy about sex, and from compartmentalizing social issues from one another. A genocidal component is also perceivable, with behavioral illnesses related to sex and gender on the increase: eating disorders, AIDS and other STD's, cutting. Freud's idea of the sexual saturation of culture, political economy, art, and beauty, may indeed be a reality, except in the reverse of his conceptualization: it is not so much the case that sex has been reduced to polite social convention, as that cultural phenomena including sex and desire have been obfuscated into the graphic orientations of male sexual desires. An example is the relations between sexual problems and the obesity epidemic. Has the pervasiveness of Viagra introduced any reflection on or wariness about today's prominent idea that a woman must wear a size zero to two to be datable and marriageable, especially in the context of the growing rates of obesity? Must she be smaller than her man's penis, so that she won't compete? What about AIDS; are the professionals who sell and those who prescribe Viagra proactive in warning of the STD's that may result from unwise uses of their product? And consider children. Enduring love for family motivates human heterosexual monogamy; this is a truism from grandfather Freud that few people even today would refute. Humans limit their sexual ecstasy out of veneration for and the desire to live with their children. And yet the abuse and neglect of children by adults, including the production of massive childhood obesity, is not on the decline. Nor is bullying and teasing, among children.[3] Regarding education, western industrial countries now express unwillingness to support their public schools and universities, and keeping young people ignorant is a form of abuse.[4] Willfully perpetuating ignorance is in fact a component of tyranny, since an uninformed public is less likely to question the authority of leaders who win through con artistry. Yet despite this absence of attention in politics and in love even for the children, Viagra and its cousins continue to sell at astonishing rates. Perhaps the purported emotive base for couple-hood, the interest in rearing the young, providing for their education, keeping them safe and teaching them good parenting and good citizenship, is less of a heartfelt collective valuation than the body politic wants to admit. As a reconsideration of Freud's idea of the death wish in the context of issues in contemporary relationships, if people were honest they would see that it is after all socially acceptable in the twenty-first century to exterminate the children in order for adults to enjoy more of their iconographic sex, as long as this can be done bureaucratically, through legislation, the media, and banking, rather than hands-on, at least when rich and middle-class parents are in the picture.

Affective justice is not a utopian dream and will not be an "achievement," e.g. a new social contract or the spoils of another war or still another storybook for the benefit of the courts and pulpits. Affective justice is a process, experienced by everyone on some occasions in their lives, e.g. at instances of community awareness, solidarity, or resistance, and it can shape the future, by transforming mood and imagination. Today's world has a chance to reclaim, to repeat and return to, but now as a feminist and biopolitical returning rather than that of modernistic sociobiology upon whose concepts Viagra was nostalgically invented and marketed, a reflection upon the issue posed in those rather sleazy tweets about "hierarchies of needs" which junk psychology has bandied about since the 1950's. Humans do in fact have a primordial need: first and foremost, to perceive that they are in this world together! If one acknowledges the truth of this maxim and applies it to the sexuality of the present day, one must conclude that the sex by numbers compulsion would actually be a form of genocide no less murderous than tolerating female circumcision and polygamy; or than erasing such sexual rights as contraception, abortion, and engaging in sex other than the missionary position even between married persons; or destroying public education; promoting STD's; or valorizing suicidal eating behaviors. There needs to be as much feminist attention to and awareness of women's sexual feelings, concerns, and behaviors as there are to fitness, nutrition, and educational policies. Solutions to these overwhelming problems must be the work of all beings, rather than, disastrously the case since WWI if not longer, the bottom-line productions of bioscience industries which are run in the interest of capital. For women, sex is one of the defining phenomena of the human being (Merleau-Ponty, 1962).[5] Sex exists neither for its own replacing and repression (as in Freud), nor is it available to reification by totalized cultural and social expressions, the one holy and exalted and sacramental place in life (as in male sexual idealism as prostitution/marriage/pornography/rape, and in most religions as they are practiced). Whether the gendered disparities in sexual existence and perception have their foundation in historical, biological, or ontological origins, is difficult to say. What is certain is that all human male needs have been focused for many thousands of years on the one form of expression that men have decided they are capable of giving. For women, the exhausting recourse to secrecy and shame about feeling desire remains, for some reason yet to be explored let alone perceived, very much alive as their appropriate sexual presence in the world. Sexualizing the world[6] is a significant process in feminism, a philosophy and politics of the heart and the affects. In a sense, women are fortunate that female sex has remained hidden, because its plurality (Irigaray, 1985) has thus not been bioscientifically drenched and parched, digitized and destroyed, as male sex has been. Feminists must not forget however that many women have been maimed and murdered because of this very shame and hiding, and also that reifications of male desire have prevented feminist desire from evolving in supportive cultural discourses. Provided they survived to maturity, women have managed as men have not been able to do, to sustain richer experiences of desire than repeating the canned graphics of themselves, albeit that women are expected to accompany their male partners who choose this way of self-caricature. One benefit of this marginalization from allegedly human sexual discourse is that today nobody sells women a blue pill to reproduce these graphics and nobody pockets the billions in profits from this aspect, at least, of women's sex. Feminist desire endures as the open, the power of having a future, and thus as an occasion for a Nietzschean return, while feminist speech, a new vernacular, can actualize a Nietzschean and Bergsonian evolution of values.

4. Assigning Values: The Discourses of Biopolitical Evolution

The plausibility of generating affective justice, that is, a new ethos with sex as a human creative and loving activity from the heart of the transformation, along with education, fitness, art, and politics, is of course the most hilarious joke imaginable among men. From time immemorial it has in fact been the only joke that is told. Imagine today's entertainment industry, absent women's persistence at uniting sex and ideas! However, the endless reruns do not constitute an objection to the coming (r)evolution! Women can laugh too! They can guffaw their way to a justice that creates some ethical standards for the first time in history. They can create lives and beauty from the joyful emotions, from exuberance, and yes, out of their own laughter! Feminists recall unceasingly that the very experiences of such insightful feelings have served in history as a justifiable cause for their foremothers' extermination. It is essential to memorialize the sexually murdered women, named and unnamed, who have gone before—and these comprise most women in fact who have ever lived. These slain deserve commemoration in the form of revitalized narratives of feminist emotional evolution. Such ritualized cultural practices are important steps in initializing political consciousness. Reverend observances can welcome a new humanity with an evolutionary capacity. In commemorative rituals, a form of biopoliticized creativity (Benjamin, 1999), women now can speak and laugh and move the world onward, wearing the regalia of a complex, plural sex, and they can keep doing so unceasingly, and not be silenced, not once, not ever again! Becoming a life-world whose sexual culture is richly differentiated, nuanced by and reciprocal to language, does indeed entail phenotypic shift and evolutionary emergence. It is time to learn together what this means and how to bring about the first stages. Women must grieve for and then renounce their obsessions to cure the men folk of the archaic anti-sexualisms, and stand up even in the face of the bullying and The One Joke, and take responsibility for sexualizing the world.

Another evolutionary option that now exists and functions is one which some transdisciplinary feminist biopolitical scholars, the most famous and respected of whom is Donna Haraway (2008), favor and in fact have begun to practice. In this writer's view however, too many characteristics of this movement befit a masculinist, linear style of thinking about evolution, an organized genetic naturalism that is positivistic and not far from comprising still another episode in popularized pseudo-Darwinian philosophy. This development is the cyborgian direction. Some scholars have argued that Viagra is in fact a cyborgian phenomenon and by using it, people become cyborgs (Potts, 2004, 2005). According to this argument, many people are already cyborgs, including those who must take insulin or psychotropic drugs, and persons with pacemakers, prostheses, steroids, implants, dentures, and the like. Viagra merely becomes one more step in humans' self-cyborgizing route. What must be noted, however, is that Viagra would be a major move in that direction, for two reasons, the first being the large number of men who buy the blue pill. Secondly, Viagra comprises a conscious and deliberate recidivism, perhaps even a sentimental one, back into the jailhouse of graphic desire, a phallocentrism so literal as to be a parody. Feminist biopolitical attention must be devoted to the fact that as a sexual drug Viagra is conceptually male. It has been researched for women's use, but it has not yet been accepted as a treatment for women (Hartley, 2006; Tiefer, 2003). Granted, this male-oriented notion of resolving sexual issues involves a gendered exceptionalism not seen in most cyborgian remedies, such as those for the heart, pancreas, muscles, and brain. The cyborgian approach to a conscious evolution offers some posthumanistic promise for biopolitical liberation. There is a grave danger though that the evolution which is being negotiated is on the cheap, as in the concepts of today's eugenicists such as Daniel Dennett, Richard Dawkins, E.O. Wilson, and their forebears of the previous generation, e.g. Desmond Morris and the Nazi Konrad Lorenz. If that were the case, the admirable goal of evolution as the revolution, held dear by the progressive cyborgians and so needed in public consciousness, would hardly be served. A cheapskate's evolution is quite likely to occur if the contemporary discourses of revolution, especially feminism and anti-racism, are omitted from the processes of becoming cyborgs. A philosophy that wants to liberate the body and its desires needs to prioritize, and to perceive itself as serving first and foremost, feminism and anti-racism. Neither Caucasian women nor women and men of color can participate in this movement if they are as always before perceived as incidental beneficiaries of the new epochs in thinking. It makes no sense for a politics that focuses on the awakening and actualizing of desire to be other than a feminist and non-white movement. Choosing the cyborgian turn in order to actualize evolutionary powers is likely to be a missed Nietzschean chance, perhaps a singular chance in the universe, to engage in durational evolution of values. This evolution does not intensify further the abject failings of the present-day condition of humanity, including sexuality. That is, it is not material, compartmentalized, organized, or band-aid structured. Neither would it involve medicalization, or PHARMicalization. Most of all would it refuse, in the interest of a truly healing evolution and knowing all the while how dangerous and difficult this ongoing refusal is, to engage in refurbishing gender dichotomies. The evolution of the future, as Kierkegaard and Nietzsche and Bergson prophetically stated, will be ethical in nature. It will comprise affective justice, and be generative, the genesis, of a biopolitically differentiating humanity, constantly producing its freedoms and its equities and thus unceasingly changing in all ways: geophilosophically, cosmically, sexually, artistically, linguistically, and in ways that are yet unforeseen and have yet to be invented from the contexts of future transformations. Laws, rules and concepts, especially the falsely dichotomous categories of behavior that postulate men's sexual fate as the tragic and women's as the outrageously hilariously comic, will be of the long past, the dark ages, not entombed but deconstructed openly, splendidly, by an archeology that resounds with melodious laughter, not in mockery but in joy and celebration.

Notes

1. Support for this paper's creation came from the Tuskegee University National Center for Bioethics in Research and Healthcare, with which I have held a half time research position, a shared appointment along with my work philosophy, for some twelve years. I appreciate the comments on an earlier draft by Dr.'s Maurice Graney and Darryl Scriven, philosophers at T.U. Deep thanks also to Will Tarver, Research Associate in the Bioethics Center, for his assistance with the bibliography. Any errors in the text and references are solely my own.
2. To wit: The English language lacks a term for the activity being appealed to, an indication of the emptiness with which language surrounds love and couplehood.

3. As this volume goes to press, the world mourns the September 30th, 2010 suicide of Tyler Clementi, an eighteen-year-old gay freshman violinist at Rutgers University. Clementi jumped from the George Washington Bridge the day after his sexual life was videoed and posted on social media by his male roommate and the latter's female friend, also freshmen. The only charge so far brought against the two bullies is "invasion of privacy," not manslaughter or murder II. Activists are trying to persuade the court to press more severe charges.
4. The Texas School Board recently voted on the contents of the state's high school history textbooks. The new books will advocate capitalism and Christianity more adamantly than previous texts. The Civil War will be interpreted as a war over states' rights, not slavery. Separation of church and state will be presented as a rogue misinterpretation of the First Amendment. Other U.S. states will adopt these books, since three conservative states decide on the textbooks for the entire country.
5. Merleau-Ponty said this, seemingly with reference to all humans, in his chapter on sexuality in *Phenomenology of Perception* (Part I, Ch. V). It is possible however that he meant to refer only to men in this passage, as the "humans."
6. Kudos and thanks to Dr. Darryl Scriven, Professor of Philosophy at Tuskegee University, for authoring this phrase, *sexualize the world*, in his comments on an earlier draft of this essay.

Seven

RED PILL OR BLUE PILL? VIAGRA AND THE VIRTUAL

Thorsten Botz-Bornstein

1. Introduction

In a famous scene from *The Matrix*, Morpheus gives Neo a choice between two pills: red to learn the truth and blue to return to the world as he knows it, that is, to the unreal world of Virtual Reality. In real life, some men are choosing the blue pill, that is, the pill of virtual sex. Angus McLaren writes in his cultural history of impotence that men who use Viagra are "deceiving themselves" (McLaren, 2007, p. 236). Any interpretation of Viagra potency as a "reality" so perfect that it convinces even the pretender, invites a critical revision of Viagra's reality as a virtual form of reality.

Etymologically, 'virtual' signifies strength and manliness. Lee Quinby, in his essay on "Virile Reality," could have left the term "virtual" unaltered because the idea of virility is definitely contained in the virtual. For Quinby, Virile Reality is "mediated violence, clean war, and computer games" (Quinby, 1999, p. 1083) necessarily producing a "Viagra Effect" which is "a union of simulation and flesh that assumes penile erection to be the be-all and end-all of sexual pleasure" (p. 1084). Through Viagra, sexual virility is put at the center of sexual culture, but it resides there not as a *real* quality (openly adopting a full-fledged macho posture) but rather *virtually*.

'Virtual' in the sense of 'potential' is distinct from 'fake' though the temptation to construe Viagra as a drug producing fake phenomena par excellence exists. Potts and Tiefer, for example, find that "what seems to be real (a Viagra assisted super-erection) may in fact be equally construed as 'fake'" (2006, p. 270). However, the Viagra-erection is not a simulation of something existing (still bearing a relation with reality) but rather the creation of a new reality. Jennifer Croissant is convinced that Viagra sex is 'hyper-real sex' or 'hypersexual reality' and that "Viagra similarly participates in a hyperreal sexual landscape, steeped in nostalgia and generating and venerating a mythical originary sexuality" (Croissant, 2006, p. 335). Croissant compares Viagra with Disneyland in which objects "are experienced as superior to their originals: safer, cleaner, more authentic and unlikely to be changed by urban development or decay, or moral crusades" (p. 337).

Some might hold that Viagra does not produce a hyperreal simulation, but rather a first order imitation of a man's youthful past and has therefore nothing to do with Virtual Reality. Croissant is aware of this argument and refutes it by saying that "if that were entirely true, there would have been no need for Levitra and Cialis, drugs advertised to make up for the perceived lacunae in Viagra, particularly the uncontrollable timing of erections" (p. 335). In this chapter, I develop further arguments in support of the virtual character of Viagra sex by looking more closely at its socio-cultural functions determined by a curious interdependence of the physical and the psychological. It is not a coincidence that the virtualization of sexuality could be pushed through most successfully in the realm of ED because, according to the European Association of Urology, "ED is probably never purely organic or purely psychogenic in origin; almost all cases have a mixed aetiology" (Dean, et al., 2006, p. 781). A peculiar mixture of the real (physical) and the unreal (psychological), the natural and the acquired, the seen and the unseen, has been present in the Viagra phenomenon from the beginning. It makes us lose hold of our usual, common-sensical notions of the real.

2. "Desire is Always There"

The most intriguing claims about Viagra and the virtual can be made when thinking about the phenomenon of desire. Sex without desire is macho sex. The macho man is compulsive which means that he perceives desire as being identical with a compulsive drive. The macho man might use Viagra as an aphrodisiac though he will always claim that he is *not*, pointing to Pfizer's commercials, which clearly confirm his claim. According to Pfizer scientists, Viagra does not *cause* an erection but *helps* an erection that has been *desired* beforehand. The descriptions of the pharmacological notices that C. R. Samama offers in his contribution to the present volume make this very clear. The drug can augment an erection but not cause one to occur by itself.[1] The difference is subtle but important. Viagra enhances but does not create; it does not even augment the desire but merely helps the erection. More technically speaking, Viagra does not *produce* the chemical GMP which causes the involved muscles to relax, but only inhibits its breakdown (Levine, 2001, p. 238). Because erections do not occur without some kind of sexual stimulation, Viagra is not perceived as an aphrodisiac, though the result is similar. With Viagra the macho man is able to have his cake and eat it too—to have the benefits of an aphrodisiac without having to admit that he has taken one.

The media rarely respect the difference between an enhanced and a produced erection, that is, between "virtual desire made actual" and fake desire with its necessary consequence: a fake erection. In spite of Pfizer's well chosen rhetoric, Viagra is "represented in various media as a drug that could increase desire, that could make you super, duper horny" (Vares, p. 327). For many, Viagrazation means dildoization (McLaren, 2007, p. 236). The first problem is the mechanistic model, which invites such an abuse. Second, the confusing of desire with sex-drive—a fallacy that is already contained in Freud's materialistic definition of the libido as "sexual drive"—leads to an artificial view of sex in general. The separation of the arousal's manifestation from the socio-psychological stimulus called desire is artificial; who can rule out that arousal is unable to *augment* desire? Arousal is just one of the components that equip the erotic place determined by desire in which sexuality is located. For Viagra engineers, on the other hand, "desire is not considered (…) and its presence is rarely questioned" (Potts, 2004b, p. 24).

As a result, Viagra "enables a man to match his physical ability with his assumed desire for sex" (Potts, ibid.). As subtle as the distinction between 'enhanced' and 'produced' may appear, in the end it is meaningless. Desire is always *present* and Viagra makes things function in the present: "Men always want sex. Desire is never the problem" (Mamo & Fishman, 2001, p. 21). In Master's and Johnson's "Human Sexual Response Cycle," desire has been included as a stage preliminary to arousal and orgasm (Marshall, 2002, p. 135). While Freud materialized desire and turned it into a drive, Viagra dematerializes desire and turns it into a virtual quality that is always potentially available and can be made present at any moment by a drug: "The assumption seems to be that if you can get the penis 'functioning' properly, desire will follow and/or simply be enacted" (Marshall, 2002, p. 136).

We should take the Viagra engineers by their word and reflect for a while on the difference between enhancement and production. Since Viagra does not *produce* an erection, what is it that produces an erection? The question is difficult to answer, but let us concur for the moment that there must be a force that is commonly referred to as *desire*. Where and when exactly does desire enter into the discussion? It is not true that desire is always there; even Pfizer scientists recognize that this is a bland simplification: "A successful erection, Pfizer scientists deemed, requires arousal, brain messages to the penis, release of nitric oxide, expanded blood vessels, and increased blood flow to the penis" (Loe, 2004, p. 45). Do the brain activities create desire or are they the result of desire? The latter is obviously the case. Then why would the brain send these messages? It sends messages because there is a desire, but the desire must be stimulated by a real or imagined environment and not simply be present in the form of a virtual quality made real by Viagra.

What all this means is that the Viagra vision of sex does not negate the existence of desire nor does it declare desire to be ever-present, but that it incorporates desire into its mechanical model in the form of an ever-present *potential quality*. By declaring desire to be neither present nor absent but virtual, scientists circumvent the existence of the soulless ego-body described by Robert Redeker in this volume. How can the body be soulless if there is desire? For Viagra scientists, undesired, disinterested, "mindless sex 'like a battery man' (i.e. in the fashion of an automaton)" (Potts, 2004a, p. 5) is simply impossible. For them, the Viagra body is not a machine-body with a techno-implanted desire, but a "natural" body that has been refashioned until it has become "more 'real' than the real thing" (Mamo & Fishman, 2001, p. 21). Using Redeker's terminology, we can say that inside the Viagra-enhanced "appliance-body" of constantly flowing energy, the drug will finally work like nature: "The user is unable to tell where his body leaves off and technology begins; it is a seamless, 'natural' integration" (Mamo & Fishman, ibid.). However, this is a fallacy because "real" desire has no place in the Viagra model. Real desire is not a potential quantity readily available within a linear script of foreplay to intercourse to orgasm. It is part of a politics of pleasure "fought out" in real space.

3. Viagra and Nature

Some say that it is testosterone that creates desire;[2] however, in reality desire is a highly contextual notion that cannot be objectified though psychoanalysis did exactly that, by turning desire into the libido, the sex-drive, or the will. When Morgentaler holds that impotence has been "misinterpreted in the past as the failure of a man's will,"[3] the "will" is not understood as an intellectually controllable instance, but rather as a drive permanently "present" and unable to fail as such. This means that the sex-drive is simply *nature* and Viagra "does not increase the sex drive" (Loe, 2004, p. 46) but merely fosters its physical manifestation. The use of Viagra is declared to be "normal" and "natural" because, according to Pfizer, the erection will "occur with normal sexual arousal" (Vares, 2006, p. 320) enabling the Viagra engineers to describe the entire process through which the virtual becomes actual in naturalistic terms. The exclusion of the cultural dimension of sex, that is the reduction of desire and eroticism to a drive or a will unable to fail, enables Viagra to become "natural" in a very peculiar sense: "One of the primary scripts that the advertizing texts rely on is the links forged between the technology of Viagra and the 'natural'" (Mamo & Fishman, 2001, p. 21). This means that we have to do here with a sort of virtual version of nature. Viagra pretends to do nothing more than help the body do again what it is supposed to do *naturally* by "bring[ing] an involuntary bodily response under the control of a pill" (Elliott, 2003, p. 83). Both will and pill are able to overcome the body and this is called a "natural" process. That this is absurd is demonstrated when, in the end, we are asked to consider as "natural" a seventy year old man who begins to function like a twenty year old. The only reason this man *can* conceive of his capacities as "natural" is because he restricts his perception of sexuality to the existing internal link between arousal and erection (a link that is severed in the case of the "unnatural" aphrodisiac). If I'm not aroused, I don't get an erection. Ergo: Viagra is natural. This internal logic creates a self-sufficient "natural" reality, which is thinkable only as long as the "natural" is not linked to anything concrete.

Viagra provides the ability to "respond naturally again, (…) it does not seem to be doing anything artificially, it just restores a function that was there naturally, in the younger days" (Potts, 2004a, p. 5). However, in the real world, "nature" can mean many different things. Sylvanus Stall, in his 1901 book for example, suggests "that it was *nature's course* to diminish sexual power in men once their peak reproductive fitness had passed."[4] Stall saw sexuality as a concrete place determined by desire dependent on age and concluded that *this* was natural.

The result of this simplification is the complete confusion of desire, drive and hydraulics, paradoxically conveying Viagra (which is purely medical) a cultural status similar to that of Prozac and other psycho-pharmaka. In reality, these drugs, just like Boehringer's "female Viagra," which increases dopamine and norepinephrine, are very different from Viagra because they work directly on the brain. If Viagra did work on the brain it would not create a virtual reality, but an imagined, hallucinated or fake reality.

Now, through the sex-drive's virtualization on the one hand, and through its simultaneous equation with desire on the other, Viagra can be perceived as a natural phenomenon. In the popular view, Viagra does *not* function like beta-blockers, which "prevent the body from what it naturally does" (Elliot, 2003, p. 83) but it merely restores a natural function. "Function" becomes an abstract category disconnected from any concrete time and place; it is virtual. In the worst case, Viagra will become a "desiring machine" taken as a drug against "low desire disorder" (Potts et al., 2003, p. 715) and believed to be able to interfere in psychological conditions and not merely in connections between a psychological condition and its bodily manifestation.

4. Viagra and the Self

Marie-Laure Ryan, in her book on virtual reality, explains that "the virtual is not that which is deprived of existence, but that which possesses the potential, or force, of developing into actual existence" (Ryan, 2001, p. 27). In the medico-scientific terms issued by phallic engineers, erections are placeless, abstract phenomena that can be enhanced by a pill. The Pfizer "reality" is not the erotic *real* place able to create desire but the artificial reality fed by a *virtual* desire that is assumed to be perpetually present simply because it is potential. Just like the gene, the sex-drive does not exist in a real and actual form but is only *made real* and actual through Viagra.

As I have shown elsewhere (2006), genes are not concrete elements but express more or less evident facts existing within certain conditions. Though the physicist Erwin Schrödinger attempted concrete descriptions of the gene as "large molecules" or "crystals or solids" (Schrödinger, 1956, p. 29), the history of genetics shows that, in the end, definitions of the gene as something "material," were abandoned. "Genetic information" was declared to exist not on a molecular basis, but in "DNA sequences" or so called "programs," or, in an even more abstract fashion, as information that is not directly linked to "biological meaning."

The self-sufficient model of sex that is not *located* in an erotic place or time, but based on a virtual model of desire leads to the loss of the self as a desiring locality. Robert Redeker explains, in the present volume, why the Viagra body is not only without a soul but also without a self. At times, glimpses of the "self" are incorrectly reproduced through the idea of the Viagra erection as a "self-produced reaction." However, what can "self-produced" actually mean if not "being produced by a *desiring* self?" The self cannot be reduced to a hydraulically efficient body. Potts is right when claiming that the distinction between "self-produced erections and erections generated through the use of a drug" (Potts, 2004a, p. 12) is blurred. More precisely, for this definition of the erection a desiring self did not exist from the beginning. James Waddell has pointed out that any questions about the self and the other "arise from my existing in a world where I am oriented towards others and they are oriented towards me. The questions are about linkage in a shared world, where fields of possibilities overlap, reform, and create fresh ones" (Waddell, 1997, p. 7). Within the Viagra model, on the other hand, desire as a cultural or socially interactive component has no specific role to play as Viagra simply makes a potential, ever-present, and "natural" sex-drive "real." This is why Viagra leads to a "fastfood technological depersonalization" (Levine, 2001, p. 241) in the realm of sexuality.

More so than any other philosopher, Alexandre Kojève has insisted on the importance of an environment conducive for the formation of a desiring self. Especially in sexuality, desire always remains the "desire of the desire of the other." We do not simply desire, but we desire to be desired because we want the recognition of the other. Kojève insists that it is by "'his' Desire that man is formed and revealed—to himself and to others—as an I, as the I that is essentially different from, and radically opposed to, the non-I. The (human) I is the I of a Desire or of Desire" (Kojève, 1969, p. 4). There is no abstract desire that can be formulated as a drive. Humans who are merely reacting to drives and not to desires simply have no self:

> Therefore, to desire the Desire of another is in the final analysis to desire the value that I am or that I "represent" the value of the other: I want him to "recognize" my value as his value. I want him to recognize me as an autonomous value. In other words, all human, anthropogenetic Desire—the Desire that generates Self-Consciousness, *the human reality*—is, finally, a function of the desire for recognition. (p. 7)

Obviously, Kojève is talking about the real world and not about Virtual Reality. In the real world there is impotence and there is the self; and, in the words of Robert Redeker, the self is "agony, battle and doubt." Any sign of potency is only possible when there is also a sign of impotence.

Slavoj Žižek, who addresses the Viagra phenomenon in his book *The Ticklish Subject* (1999, pp. 382-284), explains that Viagra desexualizes copulation because it deprives male potency of its mystique (a point that some feminists might like because it make men and women equal). Though Žižek does not point to the virtual dimension of Viagra, but treats it rather like an aphrodisiac, he insists that the possibility of impotence must exist because it is a true psychological attitude. Žižek is fascinated by "this gap, the fact that it is never directly 'me', my Self, who can freely decide on erection" because there remains a quantity of the "unfathomable X" which decides on erections. In sexuality like elsewhere, the self is not entirely self-determined, is not simply dependent on willpower or rational-instrumental procedures, but inserted into a place where it is determined by other selves.

There is no place for the self and for "real" desire as a desire to be desired in the Viagra scenario. The lack of interactivity becomes clearest through Žižek's description of a world in which Viagra manages desire: "What will remain of a woman's notion of being properly attractive to a man," that is, how can she satisfy her desire to be desired? Žižek concludes that Viagra desexualizes sex because, in the end, nothing will be left of the "phallic dimension of symbolic potency." Symbolic notions are a matter of a concrete place, they become real only through the recognition of the other. For Žižek, the man who takes Viagra has a penis, but no phallus. In the light of such claims, recent statements like those by scientists in the British Medical Bulletin, that Viagra "may be used as a personal resource improving self-confidence and esteem positively enhancing relationships" (Rubin & Wylie, 2009, p. 58) sound ridiculous.

Viagra engineers have also disliked the idea that potency is dependent upon the will. As mentioned, Morgentaler criticizes the idea that impotence has been "misinterpreted in the past as the failure of a man's will" because this will remains intellectually uncontrollable. They redefine the will as a drive unable to fail as such because it is permanently and virtually present and only sometimes not real. And then Viagra can help. Interestingly, the functional character of Viagra negates not only the real, but also the imagination which is such an important part of sexual reality. It is important to point out the distinction between the virtual and the imaginary. While the virtual is unerotic and desexualizing, imagination is highly sexual. Very often this difference is not acknowledged. Croissant, for example, mentions the augmentation of sexual fantasy through pornography which has, in her opinion, "a hyperreal quality that produces models of women's bodies and sexuality that no 'real' women can live up to" (p. 336). However, pornography is not virtual but imagined, which is—notwithstanding the mechanized character of pornography—still in the field of the erotic.

In his film *The Perverts Guide to Cinema,* Žižek (2006) points to the necessary transference of the erotic place into the realm of the imagination: "In sexuality, it's never only me and my partner, or more partners, whatever you are doing. There has to be always some fantasmatic element. There has to be some third imagined element which makes it possible for me, which enables me, to engage in sexuality." Žižek explains that the mere "reality" of sexuality can actually feel quite bland ("my God, what am I doing here, doing these stupid repetitive movements") without some fantasmatic support. Sex is constantly permeated by the unreal, but not by the virtual which is disconnected from both reality and imagination.

5. Conclusion

The restoration of a natural male function via Viagra does *not* lead to the creation of a reality. When Potts and Tiefer say that a Viagra-assisted super-erection *seems* to be real but it is actually fake, we have to ask what are the standards of reality? The erection is *there*, why would it be fake? Finally, an erection is proof for the existence of a sex-drive—what could be more real? It is real just like "Andropause is a fact, not a fiction" (Nicolls quoted from Marshall, 2007, p. 520). The problem is that reality is always linked to a time/place, which is in this case the time/place of desire. Super-erections might be "natural" at a certain place and a certain time, but they are not natural in others. The confusion of desire and drive leads to circular reflections that turn desire into a virtual phenomenon disconnected from concrete reality; why bother about desire if Viagra gives you an erection anyway? Or a Viagra consumer might think that the fact that he has an erection proves that there must have been desire. Here reality becomes genuinely virtual in the sense of a self-producing reality unable to refer to authenticity. Authenticity can only exist in time/place.

Desire is real; however, it is nothing but a condition perpetually produced in time and space. In other words, sex takes place in time and space conditioned by desire. The consumption of too much alcohol, for example, influences desire as much as age. Desire produces its own time and space that cannot not be dictated by Viagra. Obviously, Levitra and Cialis, are advertised "to make up for the perceived lacunae in Viagra, particularly the uncontrollable timing of erections" (Croissant, 2006, p. 336). The problem is that desire is never perpetual (like Virtual Reality) but the space of desire is rather a tragic land, "tragic" in the sense in which it is defined by Nietzsche. It is no Newtonian physical space that can be measured in inches but rather an Aristotelian, "natural" place subjected to the laws of space and time.

Notes

1. A. Morgentaler, "Male Impotence" in *Lancet*, 354 (1999), p. 1713, quoted from Thompson, 2008, p. 77.
2. Cf. Marshall 2006 quoting R. Werland, 'Manhood Checkup', *Chicago Tribune*, 27 June 2004, 9: "If you think you can Viagra your way out of this one, think again: It and similar drugs might help with the mechanics, but not with desire; testosterone is what fires the libido" (p. 352).
3. Morgentaler quoted from Thompson, 2008, p. 83.
4. Sylvanus Stall, Stall, S. *What a Man of Forty-Five Ought to Know*. Philadelphia:

VIR Publishing Co. 1901, p. 59, quoted from Marshall, 2006, p. 346, my italics. Marshall continues: “The author saw this as an advantage because ‘the stress of passion will be past, the imagination will become more chastened, the heart more refined, the lines of intellectual and spiritual vision lengthened, the sphere of usefulness enlarged’.”

Eight

VIRILITY, VIAGRA, AND VIRTUE: RE-READING *HUMANE VITAE* IN AN AFRICAN LIGHT

Anthony Okeregbe

1. Introduction

When an African man, or any man for that matter, undresses before his chosen companion for a round of hot sex, and he imagines the turgidity of his erect member, as he beholds the enticing nudity of this willing partner on whom he desires to unleash the terror of his phallus, a certain feeling of narcissism overtakes him and he is gratified by this gracious endowment of providence. But then, he soon realizes, having been awakened from his reverie, that this is just make-believe, a mere figment of his fertile imagination. At this auspicious moment, when the test of manhood beckons, he experiences a trepidation that often comes from erectile dysfunction and premature ejaculation, and in this painful state of longing for unattainable, pleasure his virility is being put to test.

In today's world, Contemporary African Catholics are challenged by the competition going on over which institution, the Church, Science and Medicine, should be the herald of the message of conjugal act. Is conjugal life a domain of spirituality? Or of biology? Could this be a justification for the "vast and ever increasing gap between the teaching of the church and the practice of the faithful" (Odeyemi, 2004, pp. 4)? In this paper, I intend a philosophical analysis of the resultant ethical tension through a re-reading of the papal encyclical *Humane Vitae*,[1] from an African perspective. I argue that the ethical concerns raised by the encyclical are pertinent to 'viagrification', even though the encyclical precedes Viagra. Dwelling on the same Kantian principles on which the encyclical builds its argument on sexuality, I also argue that the viagrification of sex is a physiological hedonistic pursuit that undermines the sacred and more profound uses of sex.

2. Sexual Virility: In Search of a 'Lost' Potency

The idea of putting virility to test through the sexual act is a common practice everywhere. Despite the complexity of cultures and the diversity of peoples, efficiency in sexual act performance and appropriate response to the ritualized hegemonic male-centered sexual theatrics have always been construed as the single chief determinant of what it means to be a 'man'. In her popular article, "In Search of the Perfect Penis: The Medicalization of Male Sexuality," Leonore Tiefer, drawing from psychological postulations, avers that generally virility finds its most potent expression in the genital sexuality characterized by erection and orgasm (Tiefer, 1986, pp. 579-599). From her study of several authoritative works on the subject, Tiefer delineated ten assumptions associated with men's sexual experience, which valorize men's sexual preferences, positively exaggerate men's sexual experiences, and overestimate men's capability and capacity for sex, all to the relegation of the woman's role (ibid., p. 581). Virtually all of these beliefs, by Tiefer's contention, require erection and ejaculation (ibid.), or to put it in another language, a glorification of the penis.

However, nowhere is this valorization of the penis more evident than in the racialized black male sexuality portended by ancient texts, Victorian literatures, historical and autobiographical works, as well as experiences from the slave trade. In a study titled "The Sexual Practices of Black Males and Societal Myths about Them: A Historical Overview and Contemporary Analysis," Sadie M. Sheafe (2007) addressed certain stereotypes that not only portray the black males' penises as macro phallic, but also that black male potency and virility are greater than white males. In her analysis of the myths surrounding the sexual practices of black males, she concludes that:

> Science sought to prove the bestiality of black males by using his superior penis size as proof of an animalistic relationship. The penis became racialized. The sexual libido of the African was equated to the sex drive of the sub-Saharan African male baboons whose phallus is almost always erect (...). "Nowhere was the supposed link between the African's penis and his bestial sexuality cited more often, or more insistently than in the United States. There, the image of the African slave as a walking penis had another origin separate from speculations emanating from specimen jars or the Bible" (Freedman, 2001). (Sheafe, 2007, p. 271)

But sex drive and big penises are of no value in themselves; they are no more active as an unconnected battery that is unable to generate electric current. Likewise, an erect penis is not a value in itself, for its functionality and capability are ascertained by its demonstrated potency, namely, the ability to copulate and sustain phallic mechanical efficiency during intercourse as well as the ability to produce offspring. By this token, virility for the African is ascertained from testimonials emanating from the women who have experienced the efficiency of a potent phallus. Some proverbs, depicting the sexual objectification of the woman, lend credence to this view of male sexual virility. For instance, the Igbo proverbs "One cannot be afraid of a wide vagina because it cannot sex itself" and "A woman carrying a vagina would not be asked in order to be sexed, that the vagina is her own, but when it causes trouble, the real owner (of the vagina) would be looked for," are pronouncements of the determinacy of masculinity (Hussein, 2005, p. 66). They reveal an index of hegemonic masculinity that tends to portray vaginas and their carriers as passive objects to be sought after by men who are desirous of expressing their virility by whatever means. This proverbial rendition of hegemonic masculinity is not restricted to the aboriginal African society alone. Even amongst African-American communities, this image of masculinized sexuality is relived through gender socialization of black boys. Danielle M. Wallace, in her article, "It's a M-A-N Thang: Black Male Gender Role Socialization and the Performance of Masculinity in Love Relationships," observes that an uncomplimentary bequeathal on the young African-American male is the thinking that to be a real man primarily involves "ability to engage in patriarchal sex that emphasizes conquest, and the ability to spread their seed to make babies" (Wallace, 2007, p. 17).

Thus, virility is implied in the objectification of the woman, for a woman is the necessary antipode to put virility in perspective: a sexually satisfied woman, a hyper-sated lady pumped to orgasmic release, or a pregnancy from a fecund maiden recreated by the power of the phallus. Little wonder, therefore, as Taiwo Oloruntoba-Oju observed, in the Yoruba contemporary popular culture, the sight of a dashing and powerful male tends to provoke in women a spontaneous and passionate prayer expressing a desire for marital relationship or sexual liaison (Oloruntoba-Oju, 2009, p. 6).

But beyond sexual satisfaction of a woman, the ultimate attestation of virility is the capability or ability to produce offspring. An erect penis or a turbo-charged sex drive is meaningless if the erection cannot attain its procreative goal, namely, the production of offspring. As Geoffrey Tangwa points out, "in African culture, children are highly valued; so highly valued that procreation is considered the main purpose of marriage. In Africa, marriage for mere companionship is rare, if not completely non-existent" (Tangwa, 2004, p. 391).

Consequently, from the standpoint of the black African, an imposing physical stature, bulging muscles and bestial stamina expressed in labor do not yet spell out virility, until they have been sufficiently proven by a satisfactory act of copulation and procreation. Viewed from the standpoint of sexual preference, a celibate who has never 'known' a woman is just a man whose sexual identity is shrouded in his public body. By this same token, a gay, or a man whose only sexual experience is limited to masturbation, has not yet proven his virility. Thus, virility is established in a heterosexual union, in which a sexually satisfied woman is the epistemically worthy testimonial. For a man who has been conditioned by cultural imperatives and centuries of stereotypes concerning the mythic sexual prowess of his forebears, any means of regaining a 'lost' potency would surely be a welcome development.

3. The Lure of Viagrification

It is partly for this reason that Viagra and other sex performance enhancing drugs find acceptability as off the counter commodities; concocted variants and herbal simulations of these drugs are hawked in locals markets, while refined variants are advertised in many African soft-sale magazines and websites. For instance, the herbal remedy *Yohimbe*, otherwise known as the 'African Viagra' is advertised on and is available online. The popularity accorded Viagra in the West has rekindled confidence in herbal and traditional medicine in Africa to such a point that *Burantashi*, an acclaimed aphrodisiac and penile-erection enhancing powder derived from the bark of the African tree *Pausinystalia yohimbe*, has received equal attention as an African Viagra. Every week, a Nigerian firm, Zee Virtual Media, celebrates its provision of excellent services in the improvement of sex lives on the advert pages of fashion and style magazines as well as in its websites. Apart from its advertisement in the pages of Nigeria's Fashion and Style magazine, *PM News* and *The Sun*, on April 30, 2008, this firm embarked on an aggressive marketing by sending text messages to customers. In fact, one of its numerous advert copies sent to prospective customers by aggressive text messages reads: "We have everything from Erection aids to Orgasm Gels."

Now, suppose our sexually incapacitated man in question comes to realize his predicament, and decides to pop a 50mg Viagra tablet into his mouth based on either a face-to-face encounter with a physician or from his acquaintances with some ubiquitous physicians on the internet. Suppose, then, a few minutes later he experiences some invigoration that registers in his penis as an iron-cast erection. And suppose during this short period of transformation, he is thrown onto an ecstatic world of penile animation and rejuvenation that provide stamina for blissful sex. His renewed world would be a simulation of the nostalgic sexual experience of years gone by, and which in the Baudrillardian sense is a distorted replica of what does not exist. Our man has been bitten by the bug of viagrification, a new cultural value of sexuality, which entails the whole process of turning the private biosocial and spiritual experience of conjugal relationship into a consumerist culture of drug production and marketization of packaged virility.

Thus, "Viagra-based sexual experience is nothing more than a first order simulation, one that is a simple reflection of reality," and "the drug allows a revisiting of a once-attainable youthful sexuality" (Croissant, 2006, p. 336). Having taken Viagra to guarantee that his penis will become erect and will achieve its end of producing orgasms" (ibid., p. 338), can anything be said to be morally wrong or immoral in this act? What is immoral in trying to transcend the limits imposed by nature through the use of drugs? Ought not a man who is desirous of sexual virility use Viagra for therapeutic purposes? A man recognizes his pathological situation, finds succor in Viagra, takes it, and then gets some relief. What is wrong with this? This is the moral quarry to which we shall direct our philosophical searchlight, but we do this in the light of the *Humane Vitae*, an influential papal encyclical whose moral principles condemn the artificial means of contraception on the basis of its unnaturalness. We argue that if artificial contraception is immoral on the basis of its unnaturalness, so also is the use of Viagra. But before that philosophical reflection, let us understand the principles contained in the *Humane Vitae*.

4. *Humane Vitae*: Its Basic Teaching and the Moral Challenge

The *Humane Vitae* purports to teach faith and doctrine regarding the nature of marriage and conjugal love. It begins by laying the foundation of doctrinal principles on which specific conclusions about human sexuality are drawn. These doctrinal principles are rooted in the submission that birth, marriage and love should not be considered from the narrow material standpoints but rather in the light of a total vision of man that embraces his earthly and supernatural vocation. Within this integral vision of man conjugal love is construed as emanating from God, who is love, and marriage, far from being a mere consequence of social evolution, is a deliberate institution by God to realize in mankind His design of love. By this design, man and woman through marriage become co-creators with God in the generation and education of new lives (*Humane Vitae*, 1968, art. 8). In this sense, conjugal love tends to possess certain characteristics, among which are that love is first fully human, demanding a simultaneous exercise of the senses and the spirit; secondly that love is an act of free will intended to endure and grow to the attainment of human perfection; thirdly that love is total entailing a mutual giving of selves without reservation; fourthly that love is faithful and exclusive until death. The fifth characteristic is that love is fecund, by its ordination to raise and educate children (ibid., art. 9).

The consequence of these characteristics of conjugal love is the encyclical's call to responsible parenthood, which among other concepts, entails respect for the biological processes of transmitting life, an exercise of the dominion that reason and will have over instincts and passions, and a profound relationship to the objective moral order established by God. To this end, the encyclical admonishes as follows:

> In the task of transmitting life, therefore, they (*husband and wife*) are not free to proceed completely at will, as if they could determine in a wholly autonomous way the honest path to follow; but they must conform their activity to the creative intention of God, expressed in the very nature of marriage and of its acts, and manifested by the constant teaching of the church (ibid.).

With this, Pope Paul VI goes on to lay the foundation on which the entire argument of the *Humane Vitae* is built, namely, the inseparable connection between the two meanings of conjugal act: unitive and procreative. While the unitive aspect refers to the union of husband and wife in chaste intimacy, the procreative aspect implies the transmission of human life. While the encyclical recognizes that it is not every conjugal act that leads to the transmission of a new life, since divine wisdom has disposed natural laws and circles that cause a separation in the succession of births, it calls us to understand that "every marriage act (quilibet matrimonii usus) must be open to the transmission of life (ibid., art 11).

5. Critical Evaluation

In the light of the *Humane Vitae* exposed, can viagrified sex be said to be immoral? Is it unnatural? Does it present the authentic (true) state of affairs regarding the physiological and anthropological dimensions of the sexual act? Does viagrified sex accord the persons involved in the act the dignity and respect they deserve? In short, does viagrified sex enhance the human personality? Although the *Humane Vitae* does not address the use of Viagra in sex, the document, nonetheless, harbors principles whose conclusions are relevant to our understanding of viagrified sex. Amongst other things, the principles found in the *Humane Vitae* provide an opportunity to shed light on the distinction between the 'artificiality' of contraceptive devices and the seeming 'unnaturalness' of viagrified sex. And this is what Grace D. MacKinnon, a Catholic theologian and syndicated columnist of *Catholic Exchange*, attempted to do when, in her article, "Is Using Viagra Immoral," she responded to a query raised on the issue. According to her, the query of unnaturalness ascribed to both contraception and the therapeutic use of Viagra is unmerited because each of them has contrary ends, and so both cannot said to be unnatural; it is either one is or the other is not. While the grouse against contraception stems from its denial of a good, therapeutic use of Viagra, on the other hand, is commendable because it enhances a good.

The Church has not condemned the use of Viagra. Artificial contraception is

> the intentional prevention of conception or impregnation through the use of various devices, agents, drugs, sexual practices, or surgical procedures before, during, or after a voluntary act of intercourse. Viagra, on the other hand, is a drug that helps males to overcome a pathological condition preventing them from engaging in the conjugal act with their spouses. Destroying or denying a good (conception) is quite different from enhancing or strengthening a good (as by use of Viagra) (MacKinnon, 2004).

She asks rhetorically:

> Is it wrong for a married man to be assisted by medical treatment to have sexual relations with his wife? Surely it cannot be (…). Use of drugs such as Viagra to help overcome pathological conditions can certainly not be immoral. The difference between use of such drugs and artificial contraceptives is that contraceptives do not help overcome a pathological condition. Being fertile is not a pathology. There is quite a difference. Viagra does not go against nature — it assists nature. Artificial contraception does not assist nature — it goes against nature (ibid.).

Despite the unofficial explication of the Catholic view of viagrified sex, I reckon that this position is not a well argued one, and it is misleading for two reasons: Firstly, it contravenes the spontaneity and arbitrariness which the *Humane Vitae* pursues as a cardinal feature of the unitive aspect of sexual act. The emphasis in viagrified sex tends to be on the pumping action of the man, a re-created Viagra cyborg (Potts, 2004, p. 2) who is viewed as the actor in the sexual act. His concentration lies on the contentment in a super hard, super big erection that tends to make sex a 'non-stop event' (Potts, 2004, p. 9). The woman is thus regarded as a passive receptor, who must be pumped to orgasms by the pleasurable terror of a rigid phallus. Besides, this human-technology combination relishes super-natural erections that provide 'better sex than the natural', and its function and purpose appear to be to promote penetrative sex (ibid., p. 10).

Secondly, viagrified sex, seen in the light of the principles contained in the *Humane Vitae*, is no more natural a sexual act than the use of artificial means, such as contraceptive devices like the condom. Though it is claimed to assist couples to attain optimum and successful copulation, Viagra has had the hyped notoriety of being a temporary quick fix which wears off, like every machine, at the expiration of its injected energy. When Viagra loses its potency and the once rock-hard turgid penis becomes a flabby shrunken mass, will sex life between couples still be said to be satisfactory? Definitely, no, because the totality of sexual experience has been reduced to the quick fixes directed at physical gratification. This mechanistic representation of the sexual act is a grossly inaccurate account of the true state of affairs concerning sex. Like every voluntary human action, the sexual act requires the conscious and deliberate exercise of the will, for sex does not take place because an object known as an erect penis (or its simulated equivalent) thrusts in and out of a lubricated orifice called vagina (or its simulated equivalent). Sex is a vitalistic activity; a union of life-forms requiring animalist capacity or what Aristotle calls soul-function. And being a union that presupposes vital animation, its exercise in the human species attains a complex nature that demands rational function. Like a skilful footballer's ball control on the field of play, or a diamond thief moving a diamond from a protective shelf without detection, the sexual act is a rational activity or an intelligent act "because of the hidden, non-observable, careful planning that precedes it" (Okeregbe, 2008, p. 180).

This preceding hidden, non-observable, careful planning pertains to a mental realm, where sexual desires, libidinal tendencies, and the required turn-ons operate.

However, Viagra, as it has come to be understood, does not create sexual desires, it is merely an erection pill that would require the slightest sexual desire or arousal to achieve result, thereby bringing to involvement the totality of man's being for optimum sexual satisfaction. Potts' observation, to this effect, is verily apt, when she writes: "(...) the drug did not produce or re-establish desire. Instead it operated by permitting his body to 're-program' the usual connection to the mind (or desire) that is considered necessary for 'normal' sex; in other words, he can give up any 'genuine' feeling of desire and (autonomously) decide to perform disinterested, mindless sex 'like a battery hen' (i.e. in the fashion of an automaton)" (Potts, 2000, p. 7).

In the swipe taken against Viagra bandwagonism, critics think the emphasis of sexual pharmaceuticals is on the valorization of physicality—an observable, mechanical, ready-to-act drill awaiting penetration. To overemphasize this physical dimension of the viagrified state prior to coitus is tantamount to a subtle denigration of the mental cum spiritual aspect of sexual life, where desire, thoughts and interests have a paramount role. What this points to is that the sexual life is beyond coitus. Rather, it is a complex vital phenomenon that comprises "the need to express love, physical release, reproduction, recreation, and to increase self-esteem (Bullard & Caplan, 1997, pp. 247-264)" (Boisaubin and McCullough, 2004, p. 740), which leads to satisfactory sexual life. Therefore, to get a holistic picture of sex, we cannot undermine this spiritual dimension that glorifies and wholesomely celebrates the sexual life.

Within the realm of rhetoric and discourse analysis, viagrified sex has also introduced terms and expressions that dubiously 're-categorize' the sexual act. Given the chemicalized process resulting in Viagra-aided erection and the hyped state of viagrified sex, action words like 'pump', 'bang', 'pound', 'hammer', 'drill', 'nail', which are linguistic registers of mechanics, have come to possess new meanings in the sexual universe. In viagrified sex a man 'pumps' the lady to submission, 'nails' her to the bed, 'bangs' her silly, 'pounds' her 'yam', 'hammers' her badly, 'drills' her crazy. There is virtually no equivalent to depict the action of the lady on the man. The question now arises whether these 'metaphors of mechanics' appropriately depict the sexual act. To respond to this question we may well imagine a newspaper headline with the caption: 'Four Barbecued in Auto Crash'. Just as this imaginary caption is a misnomer and an editor's misrepresentation of the action of fire in the culinary setting and a car accident, the metaphors of mechanics associated with viagrified sex pursue a tendency of reductive categorization that ontologically inferiorizes the sexual act. 'Pump', 'bang', 'pound', 'hammer', 'drill', 'nail' may be products of a pseudo-Wittgensteinian language game, yet they reveal the mindset of actors for whom the sexual act could be nothing other than a junk-yard activity.

Moreover, that the verbs employed apply strictly to male action, and are laced with tinges of violence, suggest another tendency to portray the woman as a vulnerable character and a passive vector in viagrified sex, thereby perpetuating the phallocentricism which Irigaray had adjudged the weapon of patriarchy. As a profound biosocial activity, sex cannot be reduced to a mere action on physical objects because it involves persons who belong in the same ontological plane, and who deserve mutual respect.

Despite the seeming ludocentric regard for the sexual act, as depicted by the use of rogue phrases and terms, the traditional African considers sex a sacred activity. While it may have its own intrinsic worth, the sexual act, tied to the totality of human sexuality, is viewed as sacred because its value does not lie in the act itself. Rather the value of sex is reposed in its extrinsic connection with the communal life, for that is the logical end of that innocuous mutual expression of feelings and desires termed sexual act. Sex and sexual relations are merely a means to an end, namely the procreation of children, and must be used responsibly (Magesa, 1997, p. 84). Sex is viewed within the broad spectrum of community existence and social continuum; it is celebrated within the context of marriage, the begetting and rearing of children, and the furtherance of eternal communion with the ancestors. In all this cycle of social existence, there is also the belief that an almighty, omnipresent God sustains this eternal cycle of life with his blessings (Deng, 1972, p. 30).

Philosophically, the plausibility of the *Humane Vitae* argument rests on a Kantianism that argues in favor of the intrinsic worth and inviolability of the human person. By way of this same Kantian dictum the viagrification of sex presents a reductionism that does not enhance the human personality. For instance, one of the grey areas in the viagrification of culture concerns the medical monopoly of sex economics that markets eternal youth through the production technique that simulates renewed phallic efficiency. Through their advertisements and television commercials, pharmaceutical companies and retailers tend to promote Viagra and its likes as a panacea for a sex performance problem, which is reducible in men to a physiological anomaly termed erectile dysfunction. With catchy phrases and fragmented imageries promoting a post-viagra good life, pharmaceuticals paint a picture of unending vitality that springs from erect penises and cross-sexual orgasms.

This unbridled commercialism is also responsible for the invention of the Pink Viagra, a drug whose curative properties targeted at female sexual dysfunction is still shrouded in controversies (Tiefer, 2003, p. 1). In this way they equate vitality with sexual performance, and sexual dysfunction to lethargy—all to the utmost disregard of other possible social factors and debilitating personal idiosyncrasies (Croissant, 2006, p. 341). But as Bullard & Caplan (1997) and Maurice (1999) observe, male sexual dysfunction transcends physiological and somatic sources; there are psychological, emotional and social conditions that are implicated in this ailment.

By treating erectile dysfunction only, these important underlying conditions and issues may be ignored and sexual well-being and overall health will not be enhanced. For the patient, expectations may be exaggerated and unrealistic, aided by the naive

> belief that sexual satisfaction and even intimate relations with others will be immediately and dramatically corrected or improved by the simple creation of a more rigid phallus. (Boisaubin and McCullough, 2004, p. 742)

In valorizing the erect phallus as the solution to the medicalized problem of male sexuality, the proponents of the Viagra culture are undermining, if not denying, an existential fact about man, namely, his mortality. The lesson, which the business moguls of Viagra culture have refused to give heed to, is the sad truth and undeniable fact about man's finitude. Every movement in man's clock of time telegraphs the inescapable degeneration that leads to death. Within his historical self-transcendence, man is bracketed by two terminal positions of material nothingness; material nothingness in that his experiential time-sequence begins at a point of nothingness when he was not and terminates at another point of nothingness after he ceases to be (Melhuish, 1994, p. 25). Mortality is a characteristic of life forms, and it is in this dark reality that man wallows every day of his existence. Thus, by turning its arsenal of marketization against a necessary degeneration process with such haughtiness and finality, the gods of sex pharmaceuticals are creating a false impression of the state of human affairs and a dubious moral neutrality, through their aggressive promotion of the Viagra culture. And this is a lie concocted to terrorize common sense.

On this account, the champions of viagrification are trying to play God by re-creating man into a techno-body, which becomes the ideal for all real, natural bodies. It is for this reason that we are faced with the "temptation to go beyond the limits of a reasonable dominion over nature." Hence, as the Sacred Congregation for the Doctrine of Faith (CDF) asserts:

> It would on the one hand be illusory to claim that scientific research and its application are morally neutral; on the other hand we cannot derive criteria for guidance from mere technical efficiency, from research's possible usefulness to some at the expense of others or, worse still, from prevailing ideologies. (*Donum Vitae*, n. 1, 2)

Thus, from the Kantian standpoint, viagrified sex reifies the human body and re-invokes the physicalist description of the human person as a sex machine devoid of spiritual elements. This is because "the medical (and popular cultural) myth of the male sexual body as a simple machine that operates on the fundamental principles of biophysics and hydraulics, encourages the perception of Viagra as a 'magic pill'—a simple solution—for a faulty component of the male sex machine" (Potts, 2004, p. 17). With this view the reification of the human person becomes complete, and the denial of both mortality and diversity of sexual expression (Croissant, 2006, p. 342) is accomplished through a monolithic medicalized sexuality marker called the Perfect Penis.

6. Conclusion

Although the human life which the *Humane Vitae* seeks to protect may have informed the Church's position on Viagra, the foregoing argument attempts to posit that the process of bringing forth a life should not be commercialized into a hyper-reality that celebrates the erect penis as the index of vitality. To condone the glorification of the penis (which promotes sex better than the natural) and to denounce artificial contraception (which may also promote enjoyable sex) is to promote a moral doctrine of double standard that terrorizes common sense. This paper suggests that we turn to the Africanist perspective which views sexual virility primarily as the means of transmitting life. As Shorter puts it, in the African society, "to be alive was to transmit life, to be reproductive" (Shorter, 2001, p. 94). This thinking is antithetical to the viagrification culture, with its capitalistic opportunism that promotes penis worship as a postmodern cultural value for its own sake.

Note

1. *Humane Vitae* (On the Regulation of Birth) was promulgated on July 25, 1968.

Nine

ERECTING NEW GOALS FOR MEDICINE: VIAGRA AND MEDICALIZATION

Dónal O'Mathúna

1. Introduction

Viagra was approved by the Food and Drug Administration (FDA) in March 1998 and became an instant blockbuster. During its first two weeks on the market in the United States (US), almost 37,000 prescriptions were written for Viagra (Handy, 1998). By the end of April, this had increased to 250,000 prescriptions per week (Rosen, 1998). No drug has been dispensed at a faster rate immediately after its release. More US men were prescribed Viagra during April and May 1998 than sought treatment for impotence during all of 1997 (Goldberg, 1998).

Impotence is the older term for what is now called erectile dysfunction. The older term carried many negative connotations and was officially replaced in 1992 (NIH, 1993). Viagra was approved for the treatment of erectile dysfunction, which is defined as "the persistent or recurrent inability of a man to obtain and/or maintain a penile erection sufficient for satisfactory sexual performance" (Al-Shaiji, 2009, p. 3486). One of the contributing factors to Viagra's popularity was the claim that erectile dysfunction is a relatively common problem. One study (in Massachusetts) estimated that about forty percent of men above 40 years have erectile dysfunction, which increases to seventy percent of men over 70 years (Hatzimouratidis, 2009). The incidence is higher in men with cardiovascular disease, diabetes and high cholesterol, and with a number of pharmaceuticals used to treat those conditions. Other lifestyle factors such as smoking, obesity, and decreased physical activity also increase the risk of erectile dysfunction. Overall, an estimated 30 million men in the US or 150 million men worldwide may struggle with erectile dysfunction (Limin, 2010). At the same time, there is some debate over just how prevalent erectile dysfunction actually is, especially that of a more severe nature (Lexchin, 2006).

Following on from the success of Viagra, two other drugs were soon discovered and marketed widely: Levitra and Cialis. Both have been approved by the FDA and the European Medicines Agency as treatments for erectile dysfunction. A fourth is available in South Korea and undergoing trials in the US, while several others are under development (Kouvelas, 2009). All of them work via the same mechanism, but differ in speed of onset, duration of action, and potency (and hence dosage needed). The latter is important for their side effects, as lower doses often mean reduced side effects.

Some of the reasons for Viagra's popularity can be traced to its pharmacological properties. Pharmaceuticals, especially those new to the market, can raise concerns because of their side-effects. These adverse effects arise when drugs interact with other systems in the body. As a treatment, Viagra fulfills many of the criteria needed for a 'magic bullet.' This term, coined in the early Twentieth Century by the German Nobel Laureate Paul Ehrlich, denotes a highly selective drug targeted at a specific disease (Strebhardt, 2008).

The search for, and development of, magic bullets has led to many successful medications. After being inadvertently discovered, Viagra was found to have many of the properties of a magic bullet. Viagra not only works primarily *where* it is supposed to, but it only works *when* it is supposed to (O'Mathúna, 2000). Unlike earlier treatments for erectile dysfunction, Viagra leads to an erection only when a man is sexually stimulated. When this occurs, a natural chemical, nitric oxide, is released locally within the penis, leading to the production of another compound cyclic GMP (cGMP). This causes smooth muscle relaxation, which allows extra blood to swell the tissues leading to an erection (Kouvelas, 2009). Viagra works by inhibiting the enzyme that breaks down cGMP, allowing it to accumulate and have increased effect.

From a medical perspective, Viagra is a very effective treatment. Between sixty and seventy percent of men who use Viagra report that it works successfully (Limin, 2010). The success rate is much reduced in certain men, especially those with conditions like diabetes, severe vascular insufficiency, or complications after prostate surgery (Limin, 2010).

This success contributes to the perception that Viagra is a magic bullet that effectively knocks out erectile dysfunction. It would appear to be another success story in the long line of scientific advances that have overcome human difficulties. Thus, taking a biological view of a human problem (erectile dysfunction), and treating it as a chemical imbalance, a new pharmaceutical product has overcome the problem. Where human trials and tribulations have failed to succumb to religion, superstition, social engineering and even psychotherapy, biomedical and pharmaceutical progress has won the day. Medicine has conquered another source of human distress.

Or has it? While pharmaceutically (and economically) Viagra has been a huge success, others see a worrying trend. Some claim that expanding the range of human problems that medicine is asked to solve may have a down side (Conrad, 2007). Viewing Viagra, or any other drug, as a magic bullet suggests that after it has worked, the problem is solved. Take out the culprit, and the problem is over. This approach might work well in treating infections, which, interestingly, is the area of research in which Ehrlich worked and discovered the block-busted treatment of his day for syphilis (Strebhardt, 2008). In cases where a bacterium or virus causes the symptoms, killing the microorganism should rid the body of the problem.

However, even using the language of magic bullets to describe the treatment of infections is limited. While an antibiotic may kill the infecting agent, other social, economic, dietary and cultural factors are involved in infections and eradicating them. Antibiotics may kill the infecting agent in an individual, but unless social factors like hygiene, nutrition, water and many other issues are addressed, those 'cured' will be infected again almost as soon as they get home.

Erectile dysfunction is clearly a different type of problem compared to an infection. Science can show that nitric oxide levels are involved in producing erections. But there is more to a satisfactory erection than nitric oxide. And when sexual 'performance' is less than satisfactory, there is more to solving the problem than boosting nitric oxide levels. Yet in promoting Viagra as the "first-line treatment" for erectile dysfunction, the biological dimension of sexuality is privileged (Al-Shaiji, 2009, p. 3486). This promotes the view that sexual intercourse is fundamentally a biological activity, based on adequately functioning organs and chemicals. Once the bits and pieces are in place and working normally, intercourse should work. If not, medicine will provide the necessary adjustments to fix the problem. Such a technological answer misses the personal, spiritual, relational, and social dimensions of complete sexuality. Yet the introduction and widespread popularity of Viagra suggests that a medicalized view of male sexuality has gained much ground.

As medicine has moved on from its traditional goals, it has become involved in more complicated conditions. No longer is medicine viewed as a profession focused on eliminating disease and promoting health. Medicalization moves medicine away from its traditional goals along a road that is less familiar and has not been adequately mapped. For that reason, many are concerned that this trend is a diversion with many pot-holes. But before examining the implications of medicalization, the concept needs to be defined and described.

2. Medicalization

Medicalization is a term used to describe the spread of medicine and biotechnology beyond their traditional focus on preventing and treating illness to where they are used to address areas of life which until recently would not have been viewed as medical issues. One definition is that it is "a process by which nonmedical problems become defined and treated as medical problems, usually in terms of illness and disorders" (Conrad, 2007, p. 4). The term 'medicalization' is usually used by authors who are critical of the process. 'Disease mongering' is a related, and sometimes synonymous, term. This has been defined as "the selling of sickness that widens the boundaries of illness and grows the markets for those who sell and deliver treatments" (Moynihan, 2006, p. e191).

These definitions capture many of the central elements of medicalization. One is that a problem or difficulty or limitation becomes viewed as a medical challenge. In the past, it would have been viewed as a moral or social problem, part of the spectrum of normality, or an inevitable stage of aging. For example, alcoholism was viewed as an issue of self-control, whereas now many view it as a disease, with at least some genetic component. Menopause was viewed as part of the aging process for women, but now it is viewed as a syndrome to be treated by medicine and pharmaceuticals. In the past, when children were inattentive or misbehaved, the assumption was that they needed to have more self-control or that their parents needed to discipline them. Nowadays, some would look on the same children's behavior and wonder if they should be evaluated for ADHD and medicated.

Male pattern baldness, social anxiety, shyness, depression, pregnancy, infertility, and other challenges and difficulties in life are increasingly seen as medical problems to be addressed and treated by medicine. Changes related to erection 'quality' and sexual intercourse have been medicalized also. The precise ways in which medicalization occurs will vary between the different conditions, and the conditions will be medicalized to different extents. The common feature is that while the condition may have been ignored in the past, or viewed as part of the spectrum of normality, medicalization leads to it being viewed as a pathological condition that needs medical treatment.

Another aspect of medicalization is how the focus is increasingly placed on the emotional or psychological components of the condition being medicalized. While many medicalized conditions have a physical dimension, these are not usually disabling or life-threatening. During the medicalization process, the focus is shifted to the emotional aspects. Although erectile dysfunction can be a warning sign that cardiac problems may develop, the focus is usually on its non-physical risks. For example, erectile dysfunction was reported to pose "a major threat to personal relationships and quality of life of the affected individuals" (Rosen, 1998, p. 1599). Elsewhere it is stated that erectile dysfunction "is often detrimental to a man's quality of life, self-esteem, and interpersonal relationships and is increasingly considered an issue for the man and his female sexual partner" (Al-Shaiji, 2009, p. 3486).

Ironically, however, even while the emotional symptoms are focused on, the treatment reverts back to the physical. The recommendations will usually be for surgical or pharmaceutical interventions. A man with erectile dysfunction is said to have immense struggles with depression and self-esteem. But rather than recommending counseling or personal reflection to examine his feelings and thoughts about himself, the solution is said to lie in a little blue pill that will take away all the problems. Yet in many cases, the relational and psychological problems may precede and underlie the erectile difficulties. By taking a pill, the physical dimension may be taken care of, but the deeper issues may not be addressed. Medicalization is thus in keeping with the magic bullet concept which targets the biological issues but fails to address the broader interpersonal and social context.

Shifting the type of symptoms focused on leads to a diagnosis that becomes much more subjective. Some cases of erectile dysfunction arise for physiological reasons or as a complication from using certain other medications. Relatively objective diagnostic tests can reveal when this is the case and lead to corrective steps being taken. This is in keeping with traditional medical diagnoses and treatment. Various diagnostic tests can reveal when someone has an infection, or a broken leg, or cancer, and this helps guide treatment decisions. All such tests have subjective and interpretive components, and some medical problems do not have clear-cut diagnostic criteria. For example, blood pressure can be measured objectively, but the value at which medical treatment should be started involves subjective evaluation. However, medicalization brings to the doctor's attention conditions that are highly subjective and personalized. Healthcare professionals are therefore put in positions where it is very difficult to determine which intervention is best for which person. When the symptoms are socially determined and highly subjective, they are more open to manipulation by forces such as mass media, advertising, and public opinion. It is no coincidence that conditions where medicalization is a concern have also been strongly influenced by advertising campaigns that help to create the perception that many people require treatment (Applbaum, 2006).

One of the consequences of medicalizing a problem is that the appropriate response becomes a medical treatment. "Choosing to call a set of phenomena a disease involves a commitment to medical intervention [and] the assignment of the sick role" (Engelhardt, 1975, p. 137). The practical effect of medicalization is seen in "the availability of medications to treat what until recently have been regarded as the natural results of aging or as part of the normal range of human emotions" (Lexchin, 2006, p. e132).

The types of treatments made available become important. As mentioned above, it is ironic that while non-physical symptoms are emphasized to raise awareness of a condition, the proposed treatments are primarily biological. This raises questions about whether or not people are getting the type of treatment they most need. However, the treatments offered are those that fit well with those who are seeking to promote medicalization.

3. The Forces Behind Medicalization

The forces behind medicalization are numerous, and vary with the specific condition or treatment being discussed. The direction of medicalization is not one-way. While numerous conditions have become medicalized in recent years, some have been demedicalized. For example, homosexuality was at one time classified as a psychiatric problem, whereas today it is viewed as a lifestyle choice or just part of the spectrum of sexual interests. Childbirth became increasingly medicalized, but in recent years there has been a move away from this towards natural childbirth.

Three groups play a prominent role in most instances of medicalization, including that of Viagra. These are the medical professions, the pharmaceutical industry, and patient groups. Male sexuality was being medicalized long before Viagra arrived on the market (Tiefer, 1986). This can be seen in the changing terminology used for problems with male sexuality. "The key to medicalization is definition. That is, a problem is defined in medical terms, described using medical language, understood through the adoption of a medical framework, or 'treated' with a medical intervention" (Conrad, 2007, p. 5).

A study of the terms used in the professional literature to describe sexual problems noted some interesting trends (Elliot, 1985). Between 1940 and 1970, the terms 'impotence' and 'frigidity' occurred with almost equal frequency. However, between 1970 and 1985, use of the word 'impotence' dramatically increased in the psychological literature, while 'frigidity' almost disappeared. During this time, urologists became increasingly interested in men's sexual function. Various types of penile implants and injections were developed and used to treat problems with erections (Tiefer, 1994). However, impotence continued to be viewed as primarily a psychological issue, and not a biological one. This limited the role medicine would play in treating these conditions.

Two important factors then changed. The term 'impotence' is loaded with negative connotations about men's power and vigor. Although it literally means partial or complete loss of erectile function, "the first definition dictionaries give for impotence never mentions sex but refers to a general loss of vigor, strength, or power" (Tiefer, 1986, p. 579). This was changed in 1992 at a Consensus Conference sponsored by the National Institutes of Health (NIH). Such conferences investigate the current state of knowledge in an area of health and make recommendations for policy guidelines and future funding. One of this conference's recommendations was that the term 'impotence' be replaced by 'erectile dysfunction' (NIH, 1993). Now the condition sounded much more like a medical problem.

Around the same time, what was believed to be the main cause of erectile dysfunction was changed, which also made the condition appear more like a medical one. Part of the stigma regarding impotence was an assumption that the problem was 'all in one's head.' If that was the case, medicine at the time could do little about it. Medical devices and implants showed some effectiveness, although exactly how effective they were remains questionable. These developments suggested that physiology played a more significant role in erectile dysfunction, leading to a headline in *Time* magazine about these devices declaring "It's Not All In Your Head" (Toufexis, 1988, p. 94).

In 1992, a more significant discovery was made: the role of nitric oxide in producing erections. Newspaper headlines and academic articles greeted the news as having dramatic implications for erectile dysfunction (Tiefer, 2006).

Suddenly, most cases of erectile dysfunction were declared as being due to biological and not psychological causes. If that was the case, medical solutions were of greater value. The push towards medicalization thus brings together medical professionals and the producers of medical treatments.

Much of the ground-work for medicalization of erectile dysfunction had been laid before Viagra arrived. Some men have a biological cause for their erectile dysfunction, and in those cases, Viagra is an effective and safe treatment for their medical condition. However, debate continues regarding the precise prevalence of erectile dysfunction (Lexchin, 2006). Some of this depends on how severe and how frequently men's problems occur. Studies have found that even when men have erectile dysfunction, they and their partners report being satisfied sexually (Tiefer, 1994). Such factors complicate determinations of the prevalence of erectile dysfunction.

What is clear, however, is that Pfizer, the manufacturers of Viagra, sought to convey the impression that erectile dysfunction was very common and of significant concern to many men (Lexchin, 2006). Erectile dysfunction becomes more common with age, but advertising for Viagra focused increasingly on younger men. Professional athletes were recruited to promote the benefits of the drug, and Viagra became the official sponsor of a race car and sports announcements. "While Viagra was first promoted for older men, Pfizer soon saw a much larger potential market. The pharmaceutical company extended its direct-to-consumer advertising to include virtually all men, and this expanded the definition of erectile dysfunction to include any erectile difficulties at any age" (Conrad, 2007, p. 44). All of this helped to generate the impression that erectile dysfunction was a widespread problem and that Viagra was the solution to any degree of difficulty men had. Thus, "physicians' role in medicalization is decreasing as that of the pharmaceutical promoters is increasing" (Conrad, 2007, p. 19).

The target audience for medicalized treatments is not a group of passive recipients. This is particularly the case with Viagra. Consumer advocacy groups formed in the 1980s with names like Impotents Anonymous (IA) and I-Anon (Tiefer, 1986). Such groups engaged with medical and manufacturing organizations involved with erectile dysfunction. These organizations and their educational campaigns promoted the view that erectile dysfunction was primarily biological rather than psychological.

As the same time, cultural values were changing which contributed to medicalization. These include the increased importance placed on sexuality and life-long sexual activity, an increasingly consumerist society which emphasizes immediate gratification, and a preference for technological solutions (Tiefer, 1986). Mass media play an important role in promoting technological and sexy solutions. Tiefer has suggested that medicalization gives mainstream media a way to discuss sex that is "clean" and "safe" (Tiefer, 1994, p. 368). All of this contributes to the publicity granted the release of new treatments and helps with the medicalization process.

4. Pros and Cons

Attention is drawn to medicalization by those who are usually concerned about the trends. Some claim that these concerns can be overstated. Some suggest that rather than fighting against the trends, they should be accepted in the hope that they can be shaped and directed. Others point out that other forces help to prevent the extremes of medicalization. With Viagra, for example, widespread use of the drug has been limited by its cost. At about $10 a pill, individuals and health insurance payers set limits on the number of pills they would, or could, pay for (Conrad, 2007, p. 42).

Others have focused on the benefits that medicalization can bring. Viagra is, after all, a new treatment that is effective for many men. This has brought benefits to men and their partners (Chevret-Méasson, 2009). The depression and poor self-esteem associated with erectile dysfunction can be reduced, and relationships improved. With the increased media exposure and general discussion, the stigma associated with erectile dysfunction may be reduced. One of the features of medicalization is that it "spreads the moral neutrality of medicine and science over sexuality" (Tiefer, 1986, p. 595). Thus, any sense of shame or blame associated with erectile dysfunction can be ameliorated. Even those who do not openly discuss the issue or pursue treatment may have a sense of relief that the problem is not just 'in their heads.' However, surveys have revealed that the majority of men remain too embarrassed to discuss sexual issues with their physicians (Al-Shaiji, 2009).

The removal of these negative perceptions may lead to more men coming for help. For example, around the time of Viagra's introduction, many sex therapists feared that they would lose their professional role in helping men with their sexual problems "and soon become extinct" (Perelman, 2001, p. 195). Instead, according to Perelman, the exact opposite happened and sex therapists have significantly expanded their practices both directly with clients and indirectly through collaborating with physicians.

However, it is unclear what proportion of people taking Viagra are also addressing the relational and psychological issues that may underlie their struggles. Viagra is not effective for everyone, with up to half of the men who use it do not continue to take it. "One reason is not complicated—angry and hurt people do not want to have sex with each other. Sildenafil [Viagra] restores potency if the reason they are angry, hurt, and avoiding sex is primarily due to" erectile dysfunction, but not when the underlying cause is previously existing hostility, hurt or power struggle (Perelman, 2001, p. 197).

This raises one of the fundamental concerns with medicalization. In pursuing magic bullets for complex personal and interpersonal problems, a simplistic biological reductionism can be validated and promoted. The medicalization of male sexuality, children's behavior, self-esteem, body shape, etc.,

etc. can divert attention from other approaches to resolving the deep pains and hurts that life and relationships can bring.

Erectile dysfunction may have a biological component, but most cases also involve psychological and relational dimensions. The multifactorial causes require multifactorial responses, which may not always be provided when erectile dysfunction is medicalized. Other reasons contribute to this, such as the refusal of insurance companies to pay for psychotherapy even when they will pay for medications. As noted above, significant numbers of non-responders have been identified among those who use Viagra. In many cases, men who had tried Viagra and reported that it did not work had much better outcomes after their physicians talked over the ways that fatty foods, alcohol, or the timing of sexual intercourse can interfere with its effectiveness (Hatzimouratidis, 2009). Discussions between men and their physicians about these and other topics led to more men having satisfactory results with Viagra. These highlight the importance of engaging with the multifaceted dimensions of a problem like erectile dysfunction. In other cases, more significant levels of counseling or psychotherapy may be needed. While Viagra can help to bring the need for such discussions to light, a medicalized approach where the focus is on the medication only will often not be sufficient.

Such issues are of concern to ensure that the benefits are maximized, but also to minimize problematic aspects of using Viagra. Surveys have found that many women are satisfied when their male partners use Viagra (Chevret-Méasson, 2009). However, in-depth interviews with women whose partners used Viagra revealed that there can also be problems. Women who found the effects of Viagra generally positive for their relationship, also noted increased pressure to have repeated intercourse due to "the desire not to waste a tablet" (Potts, 2003, p. 704). Other women were not as positive, noting that when their partners used Viagra they expected intercourse more frequently and for longer duration. The outcomes varied for different women, ranging from intercourse becoming inconvenient, uncomfortable or even painful.

While such concerns are not unique to Viagra, they reveal the problems that can be overlooked when sexuality is medicalized. From a physical perspective, Viagra can solve the man's erectile issues. But it does not address the underlying relational issues. If complex interpersonal problems are perceived to be primarily biological, and in need of a pharmaceutical fix, the underlying relational and psychological issues may be missed or ignored. Erectile dysfunction could be an opportunity for the couple to address these deeper, more complex issues through counseling or psychotherapy. The magic bullet may arrive and shoot down the need to address those deeper issues. Medicalization not only promotes biological solutions, it undermines the need to pursue other type of solutions and may thus extend or exacerbate the underlying relational and psychological pain and hurt.

In addition, a medicalized approach to problems looks for causes in the individual, not relationships or the community; "it calls for individual medical interventions rather than more collective or social solutions" (Conrad, 2007, p. 8). With Viagra, the problem is seen as lying within the man, not between the man and his partner, nor between himself and the beliefs he accepts from his culture. While such approaches are in keeping with the rampant individualism of Western society, they may not be the best for society. They may even remove the opportunity to address the social biases and prejudices that focus men's attention on sex and sexualization of women.

> The primary disadvantage of medicalization is that it denies, obscures, and ignores the social causes of whatever problem is under study. Impotence becomes the problem of the individual man. The medicalization of male sexuality helps a man conform to the script rather than analyzing where the script comes from or challenging it. Research and technology are directed only toward better and better solutions. Yet the demands of the script are so formidable, and the pressures from the sociocultural changes we have outlined so likely to increase, that no technical solution will ever work—certainly not for everyone. (Tiefer, 1986, p. 595)

5. The Goals of Medicine

One of the biggest concerns about medicalization is that it changes the aims and objectives of medicine, and therefore where it focuses its time and resources. Viagra is a relatively effective and safe treatment, but questions can be raised about whether it is the most appropriate way to address erectile dysfunction. As such, "Viagra is just the first of many medications that are intended for quality of life issues" (Goldberg, 1998, p. 65). Medicalization in general raises questions about whether medicine should take on such issues and treat them with the tools available to medicine. "Its introduction has also raised important questions about the role of sexuality in society, and medicine's role in addressing this fundamental human need" (Rosen, 1998, p. 1600). As such, medicalization as exemplified by Viagra should lead to reflection on the goals of medicine.

The goals of medicine are socially determined, and therefore are open to change. However, these goals also carry significant weight. When something falls within the goals of medicine, society generally views it as something appropriate for healthcare professionals to address and for payers to cover. Socialized medical systems or private insurers will determine whether treatments are paid for based on whether they fall within the scope of medical practice.

Well before the arrival of Viagra, the impending expansion of the goals of medicine was recognized. "All kinds of problems now roll to the doctor's door, from sagging anatomies to suicides, from unwanted childlessness to unwanted pregnancies, from marital difficulties to learning difficulties, from genetic counseling to drug addiction, from laziness to crime" (Kass, 1985, p.

157). Viagra is just another technological development forcing people to ask what the goals of medicine ought to be.

The most common and instinctive answer to this question is that medicine should seek to remove disease and promote health. In other words, "the central purpose of health care is to maintain, restore, or compensate for the restricted opportunity and loss of function caused by disease and disability" (Sabin, 1994, p. 10).

Compensating for loss of function requires some standard against which current function is to be compared. One approach has been to compare people's abilities and functions against some biological norm. One such approach holds that "health consists in the functioning of any organism in conformity with its natural design as determined by natural selection" (Christopher Boorse, quoted in Caplan, 1989, p. 56). A qualified approach is exemplified by the following. "Health is a natural standard or norm—not a moral norm, not a 'value' as opposed to a 'fact,' not an obligation—a state of being that reveals itself in activity as a standard of bodily excellence or fitness, relative to each species and to some extent to individuals, recognizable if not definable, and to some extent attainable. (…) If you prefer a more simple formulation, I would say that health is 'the well-working of the organism as a whole'" (Kass, 1985, pp. 173-174).

Such a definition reflects the broadening of definitions of health and disease beyond simply biological norms. This is in keeping with the approach recommended by the Constitution of the World Health Organization (WHO). "Health is a state of complete physical, mental and social well-being and not merely the absence of disease or infirmity. The enjoyment of the highest attainable standard of health is one of the fundamental rights of every human being without distinction of race, religion, political belief, economic or social condition" (WHO, 1948). In 1984, WHO adopted a resolution to expand the definition to "a state of complete physical, mental, spiritual and social well-being," although the Constitution has not been revised to reflect this (Khayat, no date).

However, the WHO definition is highly expansive and has broad-reaching implications, especially if the right to the highest attainable standard of health is taken seriously. No longer are people comparing themselves with some range of norms, or with age-related normal functioning, but with the highest attainable standard. At the same time as health has been viewed more broadly, increased attention had been paid to patient autonomy, and the rights of patients to make their own health care decisions. This has led to more individualized definitions of health and illness. Someone may be told that his condition is normal for someone his age, but he may insist that he wants things to be more like they used to be when he was younger. For many, medicine should then accept this as the goal, and help him achieve his self-determined aims. In this context, if a man believes Viagra will promote his health, defined by him as including a certain level of sexual satisfaction, then he should have access to the drug.

An older man might compare his erections to those he had in the past. One of the big challenges facing humans is coming to accept limitations and the changes associated with aging and, eventually, death. Medicalization promotes the view that all of these can be avoided indefinitely; that medicine will have a corrective and restorative for just about everything. But there is also a part of health which involves accepting reality. Aging bodies do lose some of their functional abilities. The question is one raised in the enhancement debate. "Do we accept our limitations with grace, or is it legitimate to seek technological solutions for them?" (Lexchin, 2006, p. e132).

Patient autonomy is an important ethical principle. There is much to be gained by moving medicine away from its paternalistic roots. However, as with most ethical issues, a balance is needed between listening to patients and agreeing to patient demands. The problem with antibiotic resistance has shown that when doctors give patients whatever treatments they want, the health of others or the public may be put at risk. A balance is needed. Otherwise, the implications of allowing individuals to determine the goals of medicine will be profound.

> If health and disease are nothing more than socially determined, culturally mediated and individually subjective concepts, then there will be little if any possibility of either placing medicine on a firm scientific footing or of finding consensus among experts and patients as to the proper limits of medical concerns. Since so much money is spent in our own country as well as other nations, on health care, and since there is so much controversy about the proper scope and responsibility of medicine in managing a host of human ailments that range from smoking, drinking, and obesity to infertility, appearance and eligibility for a broad spectrum of social benefits, the determination that health and disease are nothing more than subjective concepts whose meanings change depending upon political, economic, and cultural exigencies would have reverberations far beyond the realms of the philosophy of medicine. (Caplan, 1989, pp. 60–1)

Many of the dilemmas faced by health care today arise from the widespread belief that good health, as defined by the individual, is the most important thing in life. Under this view of health, when men are confronted with erectile dysfunction, medicine should provide whatever will restore their sexual function. This approach to medicine is neither ethical nor tenable. Health is a broad concept. It deals with normal levels of functioning. It also involves values and quality of life. But each of these aspects must be balanced against one another, and with other goals and values. One of the major areas of conflicting values has to do with global justice.

6. Medical Markets and Justice

One of the problems with medicalization is the way it allows market forces to determine the goals of medicine. When this happens, the risks are increased that profit will be given higher priority than the relief of disease, pain, and suffering. Direct-to-consumer marketing in the US (and New Zealand) has contributed to creating a market for Viagra and other medicalized treatments (Lexchin, 2006).

In other areas of business, this is not a problem. An electronics company advertises its product in an attempt to convince people that they need its new electronic gadget. Pharmaceutical companies increasingly take a similar approach, and begin by marketing the illness. In these areas, they initially have to convince otherwise healthy people that they have a disorder or dysfunction so that they perceive a need for treatment. The ethics of this approach are seriously questionable given the way people are being convinced they have some ailment which can be seen as inducing harmful effects on people. Such marketing tactics generate anxiety among the worried well—that growing group of people in developed countries who are physically well, but increasingly struggling to cope with the "troublesome inconveniences" of life (Moynihan, 2006, p. e191).

The connection between medicalization and markets has broader implications for global health. Market influences are increasingly involved in deciding what goals medicine or pharmaceutical companies should pursue. Underlying all of these decisions are concerns about justice. Medicine has traditionally been focused on curing disease, relieving suffering, and promoting health. However, the move to focusing on lifestyle drugs and enhancement therapies has consequences far beyond medicalization.

Private companies and public funders have limited resources to invest in developing or promoting treatments. When these resources are directed towards lifestyle treatments, they are not made available for diseases that carry serious burdens in terms of mortality and morbidity. Such trends raise questions of justice and whether those in the developed countries are taking seriously their responsibility to care for those in developing countries.

The health needs of people in developing countries are well known. People in some developed countries can, on average, expect to live for over 80 years (Japan, 82.3 years; Hong Kong, 81.9 years; Iceland, 81.5 years); in contrast, people in other parts of the world can expect to live less than half this long (Zimbabwe, 40.9 years; Sierra Leone, 40.7 years; Zambia, 40.5 years) (Rennie, 2008). Child mortality is more than 90 times higher in some developing countries compared to developed countries, while the chance of a woman dying during her pregnancy is 1 in 7 in Malawi compared to 1 in 2,800 in developed countries (Rennie, 2008).

Roughly one third of all deaths (about 18 million people per year) occur from conditions for which medical treatments exist (WHO, 2004). About 11 million of these are infants and children (Pang, 2004). In 2002, it was estimated that about 4 million people died from respiratory diseases like pneumonia, 2.8 million from HIV/AIDS, 2.5 million from pregnancy-related complications, almost 2 million from diarrhea, and over 1 million from malaria (WHO, 2004). Meeting healthcare needs in any country, but especially in developing countries, is more complicated than simply delivering treatments. Pharmaceutical magic bullets will not work on their own in the midst of poverty, lack of sanitation, hunger, thirst, and corruption. Yet many of these deaths could be prevented if existing, effective treatments had been provided those who needed them.

Other diseases exist for which adequate treatments are not available. Diseases like dengue fever, river blindness, sleeping sickness, Chagas disease, elephantiasis, and schistosomiasis infect millions of people annually, claim many lives, and inflict untold pain and suffering (Tropical Disease Research, 2004). Some treatments are available for some of these diseases, but many have serious limitations or adverse effects. For others, no treatment is available. These diseases have been labeled "neglected diseases" because despite "an ever-increasing need for safe, effective, and affordable medicines for the treatment of these diseases, drug development has virtually stopped" (Trouiller, 2002, p. 2188). Part of the reason such research is not conducted is because those with neglected diseases tend to be extremely poor and unable to pay for treatment. This takes away much of the incentive for researchers and pharmaceutical companies to invest in research for such treatments—assuming the primarily goal of such enterprises in market-driven.

The discrepancy between disease burden and investment in research has been called the 10/90 gap. The term was coined to capture the findings of various reports that found that about 10 percent of global investment in health research is directed towards 90 percent of the world's health problems or disease burden (Ramsay, 2001). Another way to put it is that 10 percent of global health research funding is spent on diseases that afflict 90 percent of the world's population (Vidyasagar, 2006). The 10/90 gap draws attention to global inequities and injustices in health research. For example, malaria, pneumonia, diarrhea, and tuberculosis are among the leading causes of avoidable death, and account for 21 percent of the global disease burden, yet they receive only 0.3 percent of all public and private health research funds (Global Forum for Health Research, 2004).

Pharmaceutical research is expensive. It is now estimated that the cost of developing a new pharmaceutical is about $1 billion, although this varies depending on the class of drug (Adams, 2010). In spite of these costs, new drugs continue to be developed. Between 1975 and 2004, a total of 1,556 new pharmaceuticals were marketed (Chirac, 2006). Of these, sixteen (about one percent) were directed at neglected diseases, despite the fact that these ailments contribute eleven percent of the total global disease burden. All sixteen new drugs for neglected diseases developed before 1999 were later listed on the WHO Essential Drugs List, an indication of the significance of their impact on people's lives (Trouiller, 2002). Less than two percent of the other new drugs developed at that time made it onto the WHO list. Two thirds of those new drugs were later evaluated as being no more effective or advantageous than similar ones already on the market.

Drug development is now guided by financial interests and concern over returns from investments. Even when pharmaceutical companies look to developing countries, they do so as emerging markets. Products are developed and marketed based on "the principal revenue generators in the emerging markets" (thepharmaletter, 2010). While diseases with significant disease burden are neglected, funds are poured into developing more drugs for erectile dysfunction that provide slight improvements over Viagra and its relatives (Konstantinos, 2009).

7. Conclusion

The traditional goals of medicine have been the treatment of disease, relief of suffering, and promotion of health. The pain and suffering caused by disease have given moral justification for social and private investment in medicine and medical treatments. The all-encompassing definition of health adopted in the WHO Constitution has broadened the goals of medicine (WHO, 1948). This has inadvertently facilitated medicalization and led to medicine and pharmaceutical companies focusing on the relief of formerly non-medical problems. Ironically and tragically, this has led to a reduced emphasis on treating the diseases that cause significant suffering and death around the world. Seen this way, medicalization diverts resources away from those who most desperately need basic medical care. Research is needed to investigate whether or not payments for medicalized conditions divert resources away from traditional medical services within developed countries.

The current situation regarding developing countries is being addressed in different ways. One critic of the current system has stated that, "the governments and citizens of the high-income countries could and should know that most of the current premature mortality and morbidity is avoidable through feasible and modest reforms" (Pogge, 2005a, p. 199). Such reforms will need to be motivated by moral concerns, not economic ones. "If citizens in the affluent countries were minimally decent and humane, they would respond to these appeals and would do their bit to eradicate world poverty. (...) and, seeing how cheaply this can be done, we surely have positive duties to do so" (Pogge, 2005b, p. 35). Pogge has calculated that shifting one percent of aggregate global income from affluent nations to a special fund would be sufficient to eradicate world poverty, and also provide $20 billion to incentivize health research on neglected diseases (Pogge, 2008).

Broadening the goals of medicine to include sexual satisfaction and relief of other medicalized problems could be more acceptable if the primary goals had already been achieved. If the infections and diseases that cause pain and illness and shorten people's lives were adequately treated, we might have time and resources to move on to less devastating conditions. We must prioritize the goals we give medicine, and the aims of our treatments. Globally, we have great difficulty doing this. Developed countries are currently finding billions to bail out their ailing (and sometimes corrupt) banking systems. Yet those same countries claim they cannot come up with the millions they had promised to developing countries. The UN secretary general Ban Ki-moon has stated that the current financial turmoil could be "the final blow that many of the poorest of the world's poor simply cannot survive" (Fitzgerald, 2009).

The banking bailout shows that we find the funds for what we value. Yet every form of justice would say that those with the most need should be taken care of first. Trends in medicalization reveal a disturbing pattern around the health needs we believe should be taken care of first.

> For in our pursuit of a near-utopian promise of perfect health, we have, without realizing it, given corporate marketers free reign to take control of the true instruments of our freedom: objectivity in science, ethics and fairness in health care, and the privilege to endow medicine with the autonomy to fulfill its oath to work for the benefit of the sick. (Applbaum, 2006, p. e189)

While we are fascinated with pills for all ills, we may be neglecting other ways to deal with life and all it asks us to deal with. Rather than seek to control every dimension of our bodies and lives, we must also learn to live with life as it is thrown uncontrollably at us. Those solutions will not be found in a bottle. Instead, they can be found in the religious, philosophical and personal discussions that have characterized how people deal with suffering, illness, and death. Such discussions have also proposed various versions of the good life, and how it can be pursued. Conrad notes that one of the forces leading to medicalization is the reduced role that religion plays in the lives of Western civilization (Conrad, 2007, p. 8). He does not elaborate on this, but religion has provided one important way for people to reflect on the meaning of life and death, health and illness, relationships and loneliness (O'Mathúna, 2000). All of those discussions and reflections are cut short when the solution is seen to lie in the latest pill, potion, or surgery. That is the underlying problem with medicalization.

Ten

DESIRE AND ITS MYSTERIES: ERECTILE STIMULATORS BETWEEN THIGHS AND SELVES

Claude-Raphaël Samama

Pour des raisons qui ne sont pas seulement
conventionnelles, l'érotisme est défini par
le secret. Il ne peut être public.
Georges Bataille

Le phallus est le signifiant privilégié de cette marque où
la part du logos se conjoint à l'avènement du désir.
Jacques Lacan

1. Introduction

The Homo sapiens' phallic sexual function is concentrated in a complexity that is not visible at first sight. It is both a neurophysical and muscular reflex as well as an application of sometimes extremely sophisticated psychological and mental mechanisms. Since the popular image of phallic sexuality is more or less salacious, taboos or universal regulations (concerning sexual needs, procreation, and exogamous laws) have become necessary, as well as discretion and modesty when it comes to manifestations that necessitate intimate contexts. A mass of abounding and infinitely variegated imaginary reconstructions, cultural functions, or simply, individual idiosyncrasies have been added to the dimension of the Eros and its potentially transgressive energy. It also needs to be mentioned that erections are linked to the hormonal cycle of testosterone and testicular production, that they become manifest through the increasing flux of blood into the penis via its veins and that this is the quasi-condition for the orgasm accompanying the prostate's discharge of sperm mixed with the prostatic substance. Still all this represents only a part of the conditions for a satisfactorily functioning erection, which also depends on heart and brain stimulation intended to provoke or support the response emitted by a desiring body (or a body submitted to impulsive tensions). Sometimes this takes place under the influence of phantasmic representations. At the end of the process, cerebral hormones are set free.

Can this hyper-sophisticated process be contained in the one act of ingesting a molecule called Viagra, which enables an erection and seemingly offers the miracle or fantasy of an assured or perennial virile power? Should the latter ever be achieved, it still leaves unanswered the status and the circumstantial response of the partner (let us assume that the majority of partners is of the opposite sex) as she is faced with his newly acquired *advantage*. If the sexual act is supposed to be carried out in a way that satisfies both, then the process risks bringing about an imbalance within the necessary sharing of desires or intentions.

The other situation, that of two male partners using the reinforced phallic advantage, also creates complex relationship, dialogue, and harmonization problems—just like for heterosexual couples. In this case, the dialectics of intercourse could be seen as forged or amplified by rivalry if not by something more harmful. The dialectics would certainly carry confrontations or the connotation of "perversity" and all this would happen at the expense of a relationship determined by *love*. The practice of female homosexuality is not yet affected by the problem of the reinforced phallic function although a feminine Viagra, already announced by the laboratories, would permit physiological modifications reinforcing blood irrigation for the corresponding body parts, which supposedly results in increased pleasure.

The commercialization of miracle products offering to influence the complex and interactive system of sexuality in order to mechanize, dynamize or compensate this psycho-physical and affective multifactual process might only be a false remedy, masking a reality based on completely different facts.

2. Sexuality, Symbolism and Duality

It will be shown below to which extent human sexuality is anchored in the unconscious. Sexuality generates a variety of forms of desire that often goes beyond orgasmic pleasure, which is potentially mixed with selfless love. It remains the vector of human life. The scope of sexuality by far transgresses the conception which tends to confuse sexuality with its manifestation: the phallic erection. Nor should the latter be confused with its ideal finality, that is, the expulsion of sperm into the vagina of a fecund partner. In reality, it carries several other significations.

Given the function's plenitude, the necessary passing from *penis* to *phallus* adds to the multiple cultural and symbolic representations or diverse preventions linked to the phenomenon. It is therefore remarkable that clinical and sometimes even psychoanalytical literature has often created a terminological or functional confusion of the terms penis and phallus though they have neither the same functions (urinary and spermatic) nor the same shapes. Moreover, they do not correspond to the same implications or investments of the body.

Only Lacan (1971, pp. 274, 288–89; 1973, p. 168; 2001, 1984) notes this difference which reflects the difference between need and desire.[1] Desire, as it is woven into the imaginary and the phantasmal, is *occupied* by the imaginary and the phantasmal rather than being their master. The Lacanian object *a* is this phantasmatic cause of the desire; it is more real than the reality with which one is normally confronted. The phallic erection and its swelling are derived from what refers, in the unconscious, to the mother, the father, and the child as well as to their projective and nodal triangulation (out of which the child does not arise undamaged). It is also derived from inscriptions encoded with metaphorical or metonymical signifiers. In other words, the phallic erection stems from a psychological element that remains inaccessible in spite of its objective causal appearances; that is, it stems from an *other* as the third instance, always depriving itself and "barring" a subject believed to be its own master.

In the collective imaginary, the phallic form first refers to conquering virility and then to fecundity through the image of insemination, but not of pregnancy, which adopts the position of a counterpoint. According to cultural anthropology, the artistic productions of most people, whether through writing or not, as well as most myths of creation, refer to it more or less explicitly and in a somewhat sublimated fashion (cf. Lévi-Strauss, 1975). The male genital organs which range, in the psychoanalytical discourse, from triumphant erection to castration,[2] are also at the heart of certain representations of Greek mythology. Here we find the castration of Uranus by his sons, we find Silenus and satyrs as well as fauns, nymphs, maenads or bacchantes engaging in love plays. Gods, goddesses and heroes are related to them: Chronos, Aphrodite, Eros, Diane, Orpheus, and the fertility god Priapus.

These characters are equally present in India as exemplified by the god Shiva and the quasi cultural adoration of the *lingam* form often symbolizing the erected phallus. The representations of this latter one—who is often joined to his receptacle, the feminine *yoni*—are cult objects even today, sometimes having temples that are dedicated to them in the spirit of cyclical, prolific, edificatory, and destructive Shivaism.

Ancient Egypt is more discreet even if Osiris is an ithyphallique goddess. The foundational myths of Australia, Africa or American Indians are not exceptions to the rule, according to which real or symbolized genital organs are presented in their narratives of origination. Invocation rites, respecting phallic power or even declaring it holy or referring to exorcism in the case of phallic failure or infecundity, are common in practically all religious or pagan cultures.

Sooner or later, *totem* and *taboo*—if I may use the title of Freud's work (Freud, 1912)—turn out to be fundamentally linked to the phallic sexual function, be it the possession of women, the prohibition of incest, castration, jealousy, or the murder of the father. The Biblical account of the Genesis, which is rather prudish when approached through a first degree reading, is outspoken about the consequences of sexual transgression (Adam and Eve, Noah, Lot...), as well as about a differential perception of the other sex that can now be seen in its effective nudity where its potential transformation has become conscious (Genesis, 3, 7).[3]

The Abrahamic circumcision invites long commentaries. Being a symbolic castration, it installs, through the simple suppression of the prepuce, a potential phallacity linked to the memory of an alliance and its divine seal. It also signifies a law and its respect but, perhaps more profoundly, it inscribes into fallible human flesh the reminder of a fideistic and *spiritual* limit.

This realm of sexuality is defined by a major emblem because of its visibility and quasi magical behavior when compared to the more modest penis; and it is spectacular when compared to the female genitals which are either linked to maternity or mysteriously hidden. In this realm, preventions and taboos as well as other connotations, divine or diabolic, abound.

Verbalized speech is no less suggestive and has words like *triquer, bander mou ou dur, d'avoir des couilles, d'enculer* (certainly related) and also that of *erection*—a medical term referring to vertical construction or to edify. And there are also opposite terms: *débander*, *être impuissant*, *faire fiasco* or *nouer l'aiguillette*, etc. which are expressions or images evoking a weapon or a scepter that is either brandished or not. One also uses the expression "*nœud*" (knot) with a magnificent linguistic intuition suggesting an unsolvable tightening or prospective dénouement. Robert's French dictionary of synonyms indicates no less than a hundred fifty expressions qualifying the male genitals using metaphors derived from war instruments, food consumption, music, or poetry, such as *la trique*, *l'os à moelle*, *le biniou* or l'*oiseau*... (cf. Dumas, 1990).

3. The Sexual Imaginary

Since the end of the Nineteenth Century, psychoanalysis has been clarifying this skein of phenomena and representations. Based on consistent and unprejudiced clinical examinations, psychoanalysis attempted to shed light on the genesis of the active genital function and to spell out what the adult phallic erectility actually is. It attempted to show that several stages of infantile sexuality precede and progressively converge until they merge into an adult and mature function (cf. Freud, 1910). Subsequently, psychoanalysis searched for these stakes, as well as for the imaginary and symbolic foundations in the unconscious and attempted to reveal its dysfunctions, be they medical deficiencies, *perverse* libidinal orientations, or collateral investments of deviant *objects*. Frequent—until then unexplained—symptoms such as neuroses or psychosis, let alone all sorts of manifestations linked to the unconscious among which the dream is the most predominant, became important issues for the psychoanalytical scene.

The phallus, advanced stage and a belated maturation of libidinal exteriorization, plays multiple and agitated roles in a comedy as it is in search of judgment, opportunities, or exits out of embarrassing or less successful situations. All this is very well reflected by the expression: "*Avoir un polichinelle dans le tiroir*!" ("Having a clown in the drawer").

The entire Freudian theory of neuroses revolves around the issue of the original libidinal and impulsive data, as much as around its physico-spiritual destiny in the psychological and "animated" body or around its sublimation towards other interests. Today the Freudian theory is much better equipped than some people would want to admit. Being different from—especially American—"quick fix therapies," which are now also well established in Europe, and which operate through a "short-circuiting" of the unconscious, and being also different from cognitive sciences and their logico-cybernetic model that will, in lack of a real synthesis, turn sooner or later towards "The Spirit" (à la Mc Taggart, Searle or Quine). The Freudian theory of the unconscious and the light it sheds on the human psyche has been neither replaced nor exceeded by any other model![4]

The sexual instinct (pulsion, Trieb) is also present as an outline of an inscripted language that needs to be deciphered and whose meaning needs to be mastered. Having to do with the repression of the unconscious, it produces—inhibited or censored—a symptomatic "offspring" that provides keys for the signifier, joining the concealed word to the mysteries of the spirit (cf. Freud, 1905). On a different scale, it will penetrate civilization and culture only stopping short at prohibition. It will be inscribed in the founding law of society and the symbols where it will have to appear in disguise to exorcise or to sublimate itself.

The theoretical work of Freud could be read in the light of a twofold articulation—individual and collective—of the destiny of instincts in the individual psyche and the collective unconscious where the *clinical* vision should never be lost, both as a compass and as a search for clarity (cf. Samama, 2005).

At this point it needs to be emphasized that the "libido," the generic concept qualifying the flux of energy and the tension resulting from the sexual function, is the available force which remains relatively unqualified. This is also true for the praxis and analysis of the physiological factors on which it is grounded. Freud himself detects, experiences, and theorizes the libido without giving details about its nature and source, even though the libido becomes manifest precisely through sexuality, its genesis, the organs, and the organs' functions (cf. Freud, 1910, pp. 120-125).[5] The libido refers either to a reproductive, normalized, hedonist finality that is, to the outlet of sperm and the reduction of tension in the case of the man; or to its transfer on inadequate, deviant or substitutive objects. With Freud, we know that the male libido is relatively well defined and that the female one is rather undetermined. There should even only be a sole phallic sexuality (in the sense of appetite and the means to appease it) for both sexes. However, though it is serving the genital organs of which the phallus is only the emerging part, the libido does not exhaust the concept of sexual function.

The latter is just going its way, it passes through foundations marked by imaginary and symbolic structures[6] that are most often associated with representations that have been deformed because of an unconscious prohibition.

The desiring subject is then transported beyond itself as it is often submitted to instances of paradoxical alterity by which it is moved and agitated letting it believe in its own liberty. The libido knows three levels and three tracks. The first is that of reproductive, normalized finality; that is, the outlet of sperm and the reduction of tension in the case of the man, which brings the instinct closer to the needs (and in the case of the woman, it is the desire of coupling and fecundation). The second one takes place when the libido is invested into inadequate, deviant or substitutive objects, which entails symptoms that are dissociated from the libido. The third one is the readiness for a dual relationship and shared pleasure, no matter if this is a temporary desire or durable love. It is not the pharmacology of desire (after the pill comes Viagra or other molecules) that will resolve (or reduce) the complexity of these internal processes; and even less will it resolve the always interactive manifestation of desire.

The question of lack, which is one of the marks of sexuality, can only be resolved through its own symbolization within a reality or a fiction that often relates to something *other* than the self. It presupposes an irreducible imaginary of which the "phallus"—which is more than an anatomical excrescence submitted to a mechanic reflex or to the vagaries of erection—most appropriately incarnates almost everything that is derived from a play of unapparent and masked exchanges. Its mark signifies all the things I do not *permanently* have causing me to depend on the feminine complement and surplus which, paradoxically, I do not permanently own either. However, it becomes manifest on the occasion of its lack regarding her, as it is submitted to unattainable substitutes that are all the more so activating.

The phallus thus proceeds as a desire where the self having an erection is as relevant as the other who is deprived of the male organ (cf. Safouan, 1976, pp. 105 and 141).[7] We will not consider here the question of the mother and the concept of her femininity, which are interiorized parts of a (phallic) desire and virility achieved through the fear of castration and the fear of the father. The phallic function comes about in the imaginary of its lack and in the symbolization of its dotation as well as its donation.

A phenomenology of the coitus where the phallus moves towards what is called "petite mort"—that is, its post-orgasmic deturgescence—would deserve long comments confirming the phallus' status of glory and sacrifice, and its being temporarily and necessarily devoted to a finality, where the laws of the species will triumph.

The phallic stimulation can proceed externally via an *object* of desire or internally via the phantasm. If the body can acquire a new condition through a pill, this means that the body can improve itself in this new condition, though still within a natural biological orbit and pinned down on the rails of an organic finality, which is then more accompanied than transcended and will not abolish the imaginary.

These succinct descriptions transcend any simple sexiological functionality. They also exclude individual overdeterminations encountered by the clinical or by the symptom. Nor do they adhere to a standardized, determined virile model escaping the random and structured forms of the imaginary which would make it *unthinkable* and irrational. The only thing that remains in terms of knowledge, apart from the individualized and empirical therapeutic deciphering, is a general structure of *schemes* that can be specified. Lacan tried this by using mathemes [symbolic representations, TBB] (Lacan 1973, p. 68–88; and 2005).

At this point, one can object that there is the "rape" where the phallus seizes without difficulty and without any reciprocity whatsoever a passive or resistant other through a simplified and mechanistic climax. However, this modifies only the economy of an act which, itself, remains dual and *caused*; it does not modify its underlying imaginary process which is here obviously woven through with cruel perversity and decentered narcissism. The latter is derived from the phantasm of a negative duality (stolen, punished, negated, and reduced to a voiceless object). *Power* is here certainly evil and inglorious. Apart from cases of mental pathology and war, one cannot really imagine a male priding himself on a gratuitous rape or deriving from it a healthy and valuable self-image. Its unilateral accomplishment is maintained only by a pathological imaginary cut off from social, moral, and personal norms. When its justification is presented through a rational discourse, for example by de Sade, it will be accompanied by a materialist and overflowing political pseudo-theory and by a social philosophy of the body overwhelmed in the name of a very *phallic* pleasure that still needs a—consenting or non-consenting—object. We can also note here de Sade's frequent use of the substitutive dildo whose only purpose can be the avoidance of any risk of impotence. It is also a confession of the existence of an obstacle that could lead to the miscarriage of pleasure that has acquired the status of a god.[8]

The erectile function that this chapter attempts to present is the perfect analysis of what is actually happening: it is a process linked to a potentiality as much as to the multiple conditions of its realization. All of these are not mechanic always permitting the inference of a *cerebral moment* that needs to be qualified. De Sade does not cease privileging the latter as a conscious and deliberate transgression. To be the/a phallus is not a voluntary act even when it can be provoked by an appropriate exercise or be enabled by a better organic disposition. It always has to do with something related to "The Desire."

4. "*Désirance*" and "*Jouir*"

Both the psychoanalytical and the clinical hypotheses show that human sexuality cannot be linked to a periodical or instinctual physical "mechanics" in the way it can be done—in spite of many exceptions—with the animal. Sexuality is not made of one whole block and cannot be described along the lines of a uniform and unequivocal scheme; nor is it a function sparked by a (medical, aphrodisiac) additive. No matter if normal or pathological, it exists within relations and within all the symbolical and signifying stakes that are linked to these relations. All of which originate in a codified imaginary.

Venal or bought love enters the same category and realizes itself in a duality. The whore affirms the significance of the phallus within the realm of the phantasmic or of the reestablished *other*. What changes is only the framework of respective intentions as it becomes more contractualized. The Viagra-reinforced and better assured male erection could here be justified through an exercise of hygiene and the facilitation of relaxation without assuming the personal necessity of another finality.

Individual sexuality that excludes mating is only a narcissistic and falsely autonomous form of sexuality. It presupposes another imaginary, simulative duality and often the convocation of the opposite sex in the phantasm or, in homosexuality, its inversion in the figure of the same. Masturbatory practices—beyond the physiological relief that they can bring—include the cause of an *alterity* in their accomplishment, of a self getting an orgasm through a virtual other.

It becomes clear that the human phallic function fuses in itself a multiplicity of factors, of stakes and of representations. This is how one can understand why so many things depend on it: a series of circularly related regulations, internal balances, images of the self linked to the confidence of an accomplished virility and its gratifying consequences, but also those images that are reflected as they are received and sent back by a partner.

One cannot insist enough that this phallic function distinguishes the human from the animal, which is only submitted to physic-chemical determinations and to natural, exact cycles of instinctual mechanisms where, apart from a specific and differential etiology, the triumph of reproductive laws and the conservation of the species dominate. Nor can the difference between the feminine genital biology that is submitted to a long cycle of monthly ovulation be ignored because it is extremely different from that of the male biology with its permanent testicular production which, in the case of the slightest process of aging, creates the often pressing need of ejaculation. This m/f imbalance represents a major difference in the genital cycles, their regulation, and their satisfaction.

If one adds to this the fact that female genital satisfaction—finally experienced as the imaginary cause or the real objective of the phallic reality as erectile power—is to a large extent linked to the penetrating functionality of the phallus and is a simultaneous cause and effect of its own desire (or intention), one can more easily grasp the essence of this very specific function. It can be concretely identified when looking at features which, apart from their anatomico-physiological and hormonal bases, are related to mental instances that spark desire beyond the swelling disposition, no matter if the latter is reinforced or organically reassured.

The masculine desire must be related to its components, which are not limited to the cause and its effect—a stimulus and its reaction—but work rather like a reaction from one "black box" to another, and where the circuits of desiring, which are double and reciprocal when they have to meet, cross the other level of what is called phantasmatic.

These two forms are different from that of the animal in terms of sophistication and individual psychological determination. They are linked to various infantile conditionings and personal histories of organo-libdinal genesis. They are also linked to various ancient traces of pleasure or unpleasure as well as to conditionings and precocious identification. They can depend on—imaginary or non-imaginary—favorable associations that can activate and not only make the erectile stimuli of the penis (and why not the clitoris [cf. Freud, 1910, pp. 128ff] easier (even though the scenario cannot be transposed in terms of functional finality) but also, of course, provide a specific amount of appreciation and reciprocity.[9]

The question of whether the clitoris is a wasted penis or the remnant of an organ that used to be better developed in earlier stages of evolution leaves unanswered all questions about its differentiated or interpreted cultural representation (we only need to mention the excision, which is still practiced in several African countries), as well as all questions about its finality and functionality. Being an equally erectile organ, it contributes to the woman's pleasure, indirectly facilitating or accompanying her desire. Interpreted like this, as a substitute for the real or the phantasmic and as producing a situation of rivalry or *confrontation*, the clitoris is not necessarily *useful* for phallic penetration! Would it thus be an obstacle for the reproductive function (which is what the barbarous idea of excision suggests)? However that may be, within the feminine imaginary the clitoris is linked to a virtual phallicity. And in its reality it is linked to a source of excitation complementary to vaginal receptivity.

In this respect, the clinical discourse of the female orgasm distinguishes between "vaginal" and "clitoral" women, with respect to the research on how women obtain an orgasm. This discourse increases the theme of an acceptable or proclaimed cleavage within the reproductive function situated between pleasure and fecundation, between gratuitousness of the sexual act and its *natural* finality. Today, the abolishment of any norm in this realm, the transgression of natural imperatives, the mastering of bodily cycles and processes (pills, suppressed menstruations, artificial fecundation, transsexuality, assisted virility, sex-toys [cf. Dortier, 2008]) as well as the wonders of chemistry and of laboratories working on quasi-anthropological mutations—all these things undermine what was once perceived as a seal of nature.

In parallel, another study should be undertaken on the effects of the (erectile?) stimulation of the woman. It would also entail, without any doubt, a discussion of interactive problems, exactly as I have shown above for the case of the man. It would take place somewhere between the apparently masterable complicity of the body and phantasms linked to other components: the acceptance of intercourse, the reciprocity of the orgasm, and the implicit requirements made to an active (or activated) partner.

The phantasm of autonomy in the realm of sexuality and the narcissism by which it can be accompanied, would, in most cases, certainly come up against a psychoaffective, relativizing that brings the intrinsic power of any kind of stimulation into play. The latter aims rather at an instauration of the physical predisposition in order to meet a *better* phallic condition; that is, it links pleasure to a paradoxical dispossession of the self. The "phallus," owned or not owned, remains for the man and for the woman—though their autonomies are different—the sign of a third instance emerging between both, an instance that they create, dote themselves with, receive or enjoy (jouissent) in the form of a transitive action and a paradoxically *exterior* object. Only the analysis of the "phantasmatic" aspect of its functioning can lead to an understanding of the mechanisms that make it present. Only this analysis can show its place, within the economy of the male, as a virtual presence and the female as an absence and a lack needing to be filled.

The Viagra for women is ready for commercialization. This product does not undermine the above explanations. The imaginary and symbolical psychological overdetermination of human sexuality is linked to desire, which is a highly *spiritual* process, both woven with the fibers of the consciousness it has of itself and supported by its unconscious weft. A *complete* and satisfying culmination can exist only on the condition of an encouraged desire and on the condition that the living and desiring "object" agrees to be a desiring subject and is, in turn, recognized as desirable and as desiring.

Without this complex process there is only animal-like satisfaction. The thesis suggesting to stop here and to qualify this as the first regulating function of human sexuality would not only make a conservative assessment, but it would also not respond to the completeness of the definition and demands of sexuality. Defined like this, sexuality reduced to needs that are unrelated to psychological, affective, energetic dimensions that increase its importance ends up as an impossibility, impotence, or as a lived *denaturation*! Clinical sexology is full of such examples (cf. Hesnard, 1959; Held, 1979, ch. 2 and 4).

Normal and accomplished sexuality can only desire *somebody*—an individual of the opposite sex—with whom she can satisfy or not satisfy her desire to mate. The acceptance or refusal of another person to carry out this act thus implies that there are two free subjectivities. It is easy to predict the problems which arise when the desire is unilateral. The synchrony of desires is the affliction of married couples and all the more among unmarried couples.

The objection of the clash of desires or their complementarities through the peculiar or even "perverse" idiosyncratic phantasms—eventualities represented by sadism, masochism, voyeurism, fetishism, etc.—would not contradict the thesis that what is at work here is a mentalism. The thesis reinforces even more the dual, dialectical, and complementary character of love partnership.

This can even be used as a description in terms of a fight for recognition, more and more frequent among couples confronted with the feminist ideology (cf. Butler, 2010; Dorlin, 2008; as well as American gender studies in general), where new mentalities contest older representations. The Hegelian scheme of the dialectical combat between master and slave (cf. W. F. Hegel, 1939, p. 154ff [vol. 1 B]) fully functions here, except that the pressing possession of the phallus can only be part of an irreversible transaction that remains solvable in the identification of irreducible selves, each indispensable to the other and a priori without status of exchange. The increase of the virility of a single partner through one product or the other leaves the process of accomplishment untouched, be it through a script or through an imaginary scene played by two—real or unreal—characters.

This evokes, in a liminary fashion, homosexual or lesbian relationships asking for special treatment when it comes to the place and the role of the phallus (where the taking of erectile stimulators is important) within the relationship. Those relationships, in whatever form, remain linked to questions of desire,[10] reciprocity, synchrony, convergence (or non-convergence) of phantasms, and the eventual partition of pleasure that no unilateral reinforcement of the erectile function can avoid.

It is, of course, always possible to object that the erectile function can be negotiated or "administered" together, made to order, etc. Such examples refer back to the mutual arrangements in a couple, the practices, the sexual affinities, and, of course, the shared phantasms. In other words, they refer to the psychologization of the relationship rather than to its psychological penchant and its support by a supplementary organic facilitation.

It is in these cases of relational patterns—that will be added to the clinical cases—that the ingestion of products can better be justified or legitimated. It can be justified not from a moral point of view, which has little to do with the often fantasmatic, interested, egoistic demands or those that are linked to individual phantasms of erotism. But it can be justified from the point of view of authenticity and respect or at least the requirements for a successful relationship that is fundamentally *dualized* in its profound nature.

5. Viagra, the False Panacea

By discovering the mechanisms that can facilitate the male partner's erection in a love relationship (e.g. the inhibition of the phosphodiesterasis type 5 and eliminating the blockage of Cgmp [cyclic guanosine monophosphate] which is a sexual product for the penis), molecular chemistry seems to propose sexual intercourse in entirely new terms. Many assume that it will only enrich the intercourse by adding a supplementary perspective that will not change anything about its essence, its finalities, the complexity of its process, and its ideal accomplishment. I insist that, though this possibility enriches the sexual intercourse by adding a supplementary perspective, it does not change anything about its essence, its finalities, the complexity of its process, and its ideal accomplishment.

The pharmaceutical notice of another product permitting a better erection, Cialis, whose product *Tadalafil* helps to relax the blood vessels of the penis in order to improve the erective function, provides this indication: "It is important to know that Cialis has no effect without sexual stimulation. You and your partner have to engage in preliminaries exactly as you would do when you don't take drugs for an erectile dysfunction."[11]

Taking the product does not change anything with regard to the necessary succession of intercourse phases, that is, the acceptance of the relation, obligatory preliminaries, and ulterior reciprocity of stimulations as necessary conditions of a smooth unfolding of the act. In other words, the ingestion of a medicine does not create the desire. It is supposed to wait for the emergence of desire in order to become not only active, but also to accompany a process that is almost independent of its biological stimulation or simply linked to the stimulation through peculiar devices that de-physiologize the process in order to subjectivize it.[12]

The mechanism of the phallic erection is that of a blood influx into the "hollow body," which is the muscle of the penis. This influx is not directly due to the ingested molecules of Viagra or similar drugs, but depends rather on the process linked to desire as a mentalized or anticipated representation, which is, as has been shown above, *phantasmatic*. It is only when all other conditions, whose relative sophistication has been sketched above, come together, that the expected effect will facilitate the achievement.

Does this mean that these products are useless or inefficient? Of course not. They play a supportive role in activating sexuality, a process that neither creates nor exhausts sexuality. The therapy of erectile dysfunction can be interesting in the sense of giving self-confidence back to the man regarding the virile image symbolized by his erections.[13] Still it needs to be pointed out that this *therapy* confronts us with the question of its own cause and the reasons for the instructions it issues. The therapy can be of a physiological kind (concerning the process of aging, lack of libidinal appetite, malformation, accident), but first of all, and in most cases, the therapy will have a psychological function concentrating on defects or embarrassments within the love relationship.

There are the synergetica or synchronic gaps of both corporeal physiologies and metabolisms (menstruation, temporary tiredness, sleep). Also, the stimulation of *one* partner can only lead to isolation if the other partner does not enter the game or evades. The offer of *virile* reinforcement can certainly be stimulative, but it does not abolish the condition of a necessary reciprocity of the sexual welcome. The conflux or the divergence of individual phantasms within couples (and today perhaps also the encounter of diverging mentalities and respective ideologies), has been explained above. It is also true that this corrective therapy can reinforce one's own desire for the partner through personal phantasms during intercourse. The therapy presupposes thus an acceptance and recognition of the sexual difference and its assumption. The *treatment* has finally the therapeutic function—when all other conditions are fulfilled—to permit the correct accomplishment of sperm emission because it is more sustained and stricter. It is adequate to a will to reproductive fecundation.

I will not enter into the question of the sexual difference and the genesis of the male and female genital functions on which psychoanalytical theory has ruled through its clinical discourse rather than through dogma, even though other things have been affirmed. The *penisneid* and its impact on the female unconscious is, for most psychoanalysts, at the center of the female castration complex and the neuroses that can follow from it. This remains true from K. Abraham to K. Horney (1967, pp. 30-40). The female clitoris is often presented as an atrophie and a lack of what the man has and of which the woman is jealous.

We need to ask if the female accomplishment of the act remains dependent on the phallic instance. Here the representations, the theory, and the clinical discourse leave the psychophysiological process leading to the female orgasm in suspense as a separable, independent phenomenon. The thesis of female sexuality and its modes of acquiring orgasms as a dark continent (a "hole") have already been evoked. In any case, this process often remains linked to a phantasmatic regime that obviously cannot exclude the father figure and phallic reality. The feminist (or lesbian) thesis of an orgasm beyond material phallic reality (or its phantasmal or non-phantasmal presentation) does not raise questions about the imaginary or about the causal power of the (similar or different) *other*.

The (phallic) images of the mother and the father of both sexual partners will create cross-relationships within a play including six players, that is, three more than in the Oedipal trio.[14] These images are fundamental even if they are not directly present in the intercourse relation. They are phantasmatically called upon (or unconsciously active) through representations and they *cause desire*. The whole constellation can be thought through Lacan's notions of the "barred ego" or the "object a" as entities that are never fully present and cannot be fully signified.

Freud sustains the theory of a unique phallus as the organ of sexual pleasure (*jouissance*). Lacan has worked out an underlying symbolic order in the modality of the lack and makes of the phallus a sort of *transactional* and paradoxical organ of the other. In fact, the phallus is not a well defined and permanent organ (an anatomically transformed penis), but a potentiality that refers to the desire which needs to be distinguished from the demand and the need. The latter two processes and the state they create are related, the first to a psychological and unconscious phenomenon, the second to a physiological state (for example the hormonal marks). The desire maintains itself only through the imaginary and phantasms which animate a complex, inventive—sometimes delirious and archaic—scenery.

In this chapter, which attempted to spell out what is implicit in the phenomenon of Viagra, I want to insist on three points. The first concerns the planetary success of a consumer product that functions as a substitute; the second concerns the unexpected resistance to think about Viagra and its stakes; and the third concerns perpetual psycho-anthropological data.

Concerning erectile stimulators, it is important to note an extremely intensive activity linked to the legal or illegal sale of products promising erection on tens of thousands of internet websites.[15] Those sites boast about all advantages of the triumphing power of the phallus for all males of the planet. Such an infatuation proves the speculative lucrativity of pharmaceutical laboratories around the need of physical and spiritual balance; but it also shows that there is a demand flowing out of the attested inability to express and to assume masculinity; and this demand results from the loss of an imaginary that has been reduced to the spectacle of a forced performance that is, in turn, the result of the current postmodern renunciation of natural virility (cf. Zemmour, 2006).

It also needs to be emphasized in this study how much the search for consequences of such products often are not taken into account by researchers, practitioners, sexologist or psychoanalysts although they topple common certitudes, dogmas, and representations of virility or of femininity as the causes or effects of sexual desire and their biological and existential involvements. Certainly, some of them prescribe Viagra and their prescriptions remain medicalized and are not officially accessible. Still, it remains a fact that the psycho-relational and socio-cultural consequences, or those consequences of potential upheavals touching upon sacred or profane representations of sexuality, have not really been approached by analysts. They will fear—paradoxically or legitimately—a competition within their own sphere of influence.

We cannot come back to the hesitations even uttered by Freud concerning biological chemistry supporting sexual processes and the maintenance of the libido. For a while they have been pushed into the background by incontestable scientific and medical advancements that would have satisfied the father of the theory of the unconscious. On the other hand, those findings invalidate neither his theory of the libido as an essential hypothesis of the understanding of psychological life and human desire (cf. Freud 1910, p.125ff; Laplanche & Pontalis 1967, pp. 224-225), nor, of course, those of the unconsciousness of the universal backdrop of any "consciousness" or that of the "ego-libido" (which should not be confused with the hormonal mark or the blood flow). It is, however, represented by everybody's parental history, by the structures of the psyche, by a blind destiny of the sex drive or, to use another term, by their "imaginal" faces.[16] This latter term—borrowed from the Persian Neo-Platonic school and Henry Corbin (French translator of Sohrawardi)—refers to the transcendental capability of the human subject, and to the subject's (logical or non-logical) constructive mental faculty and its virtual aptitude of inventive imagination.

The phenomenality of the imaginary of the desire does not create only arbitrary figures or poetical images but rather effects of vital and subjective phantasmatization. These effects remain linked to a constitutive human impulse moved by a Schopenhauerian "will to live" for which any prosthesis is always inessential. Also sex has to do with this.

6. Conclusion

The present study has attempted beyond a universal and shared experience, to assure psychoanalysts not of the perennity of their respective art, but of human sexuality and the metamorphosing adventures to which it is submitted. They encounter sexuality through new modalities and new perspectives, but they leave its diverse manifestations in the state of a naked truth. Sexuality, on its own or accompanied, manifest or hidden, is always linked to a broader meaning into which it is included. It belongs to a "parole" by which it is moved in a way different from the way in which it thinks of itself. In adult or non-adult sexuality, the spirit is not separated from the body, even though it may sometimes look otherwise (cf. Freud, 1915, p. 65ff).

Translated from the French by TBB

Notes

1. Laplanche and Pontalis (1976, pp. 311–12) insist on a certain ambiguity when attempting to clarify what constitutes an operational psychological field beyond the organ itself.
2. Psychoanalytical discourse should distinguish more precisely and more often between the penis and the testicles.
3. Cf. Old Testament, *Genesis*, 3, 7: "Then the eyes of both were opened, and they knew that they were naked. And they sewed fig leaves together and made themselves loincloths." English Standard Version.

4. Michel Onfray's book *Le Crépuscule d'une idole: L'affabulation freudienne* (2010), for example, is an exercise in aggressive and sometimes projective "deconstruction," operating more *ad hominem* than *ad teoriam* and certainly the result of an absence of experience as an analyst. In this demagogic and ridiculously iconoclastic work, suffering from structural and experimental incoherence, the Freudian corpus is constantly submitted to a suspicious malice; and all this is done in the name of a philosophical position naively qualified as autonomous.
5. Even though Freud recognizes the limits of proven scientific knowledge of his time (hormones would be discovered later) he does not compromise the processes and the clinical effects of his discovery. It is known that he rejected, for example, Jung's explanations of the libido.
6. See Lacan, 1971and 2005. The latter work is extremely rich in geometrical figures and Borromean knots testifying to Lacan's ambition to wrench psychological or other significant phenomena from their biological penchants or from those of affective psychology and their pity for the ego. Lacan submits psychological phenomena to their imaginary processes because only they enable general and exact formalization. He clarifies psychological phenomena by pointing to generative structures and by using a meta-language showing the relationships between the real (material), the symbolic, and the imaginary without letting any of those win over the other.
7. Safouan's view joins the Lacanian idea of "love as an impossibility" (*amour comme impossible*), which is submitted to this inevitable play of multiple and invisible mirrors offering its images.
8. See Chapter 6 of de Sade's *Philosophy in the Bedroom*, entitled "French People, One More Effort if you want to be Republicans." See also Lacan 1973 on de Sade ("Kant avec Sade").
9. These two features are not always excluded from animal life where they adopt, however, other proportions. There are, for example, the "love parade," rivalry between males, and seduction; but the instinct and the law of survival of the species dominate and will always triumph.
10. Literature is a pertinent field when trying to grasp the conscious and formulable scope of desire beyond the unconscious sources or its transgressive forms. With regard to homosexuality, this is true from Verlaine to Cocteau or Gide, but especially for Jean Genet, who makes the "perversity" of love between men sublime or angelic and for whom the question of virile sex refers as much to the real (material) object as to its incarnated or dreamt *désirance* that is splitting the self. See Genet 1948.
11. See the report of the European Medicine Agency, which indicates in 1988 (the year Viagra was authorized in Europe) that "sexual stimulation is required if Viagra is supposed to be efficient."
12. One could say that this mechanism concerns, through the polysemy of the vocabulary, the heart as the nerval center of blood circulation and as the metaphorical seat of emotions and sentiments.
13. On the question of the entirety of ancient modes and modes that evolved out of the relation between the couple and its counterpart see E. Badinter, 1986.
14. This sort of "mathème," which includes six virtual characters or more and not only two, has a lot to do with the dialectic of desire. The question of homosexuality and lesbianism remains linked to it. Mother and father with whom one identifies

(either by accepting or by rejecting their ideals) form a structural basis. They meet the partner's parents as models and references in the phantasm or in the ideal intercourse in a symmetrical fashion. These uncontrolled plays strongly determine the imaginary of the desire: they welcome it on an invisible stage where an – until here – unwritten play unfolds, no matter if the conditions are natural or artificial.

15. In 2010, Google shows 56 million search entries for Viagra but only 350,000 for aspirin.
16. See. G. Durand 1984. From this current, I want to retain here only the creative dynamics of the imagery and not the author's conclusions about an uncertain and profuse "archetypology."

Eleven

AMERICA AND VIAGRA OR HOW THE WHITE NEGRO BECAME A LITTLE WHITER: VIAGRA AS AN AFRO-DISIAC

Thorsten Botz-Bornstein

1. Viagra Cinema

Television commercials and advertisements have strongly contributed to Viagra's commercial success. Since direct-to-consumer advertising of pharmacological products is permitted in the USA, we have had frequent opportunities of reviewing the nation's sexual consciousness and its ideas about masculinity via Viagra advertisements. Employing, during a first phase, mainly elderly couples, Viagra advertisements quickly shifted to depicting younger men who were featured alone and employed and even featured celebrities or sports heroes. Many might hold that watching a Viagra clip is an experience closest to the Freudian uncanny because there is an always-present degree of obscenity (your children might ask "what does this man need this drug for?") is safely contained in a universe of unquestionable familiarity and civilization. Any suspicion that this drug could be used by men unable to handle it on an ethical level is decisively ruled out by the marketing rhetoric. The official image of Viagra users is that of happy, progressive, liberal, and technology-invested citizens who have made a small step towards immortality.

An intriguing fact is the quasi absence of black people from these commercials. Though in more recent times, Cialis and Levitra staged African Americans in some of their television advertisements. According to Meika Loe, the Pfizer concern was apparently eager to associate its product with predominantly "white, male, heterosexual, middle-class or above" men (Loe, 2004, p. 192). Vares holds that "in the US print and television advertisements associated Viagra with romance between heterosexual, mostly white couples in their 40s, 50s and 60s" (2006, p. 317). The TV hymn "Viva Viagra" draws on a country western theme and not on a rap song. Though two black people play in the band and sing, the music is obviously "white music" and the presence of black people in this band might strike many as strange. A television ad featuring soccer star Pele, telling people that he doesn't need Viagra, but if he did, he'd take it, was not released in the US but in Latin America (Loe, p. 185). As a cultural and a medical phenomenon, the Viagra body is clearly the normal, white, middle-class body. J. Perkinson (2002, p. 173) has shown that in the US, norms of the white middle-class body "are largely unconscious and inarticulate. They tend to encode technologies of normativity that do not require the work of conscious performance. They constitute an unproblematic physicality in the body politic."

There is a simple way of explaining the quasi exclusion of black people from Viagra commercials. Cornel West holds that "black sexuality is a taboo in America principally because it is a form of black power over which whites have little control" and that "the visible manifestations evoke the most visceral of white responses, be it one of seductive obsession or downright disgust" (West, 2001, p. 125). In the period following slavery, in minstrel shows, "even as a joke, an image of black male sexual potency would prove too threatening" (Giles, 1995, p. 64), which yielded to the white tendency to epitomize black "hypersexuality [as being] driven by some racially coded instinct" (Sharpley-Whiting, 2003, p. 410). Very early, whites were identified with rationality while peoples of color were associated with the body (Takaki, 1979, p. 13) and in the American imaginary "black culture became shorthand for unrepressed masculinity" (Leland, 2005, p. 88). Impotence, on the other hand, was understood culturally as a white man's problem (McLaren, 2007, p. 253).

It would no doubt have been undesirable to have the "myth of the African American man as sexual aggressor or 'rapist'" (Frankenberg, 1993, p. 76) reappear in Viagra commercials, even in the most suppressed and suggestive form. Though we know that theoretically, Viagra can be used by *any* man—black or white—in Viagra marketing it has been important to not compromise its positive, family-oriented image and to not address those myths that are hidden in the national subconscious.

There is also a more complex way of explaining the quasi absence of blacks in the commercials. Viagra is supposed to show us the way into a bright future and in this futuristic, science-imbued world there has never been much space for black people. The prosthetic and cyborgian[1] connotations that cling to the drug invite us to read the Viagra clips like short science fiction movies, in which case the quasi-absence of black people will not come as a surprise. Barbara Omolade explains that, by principle, science fiction films exclude blacks from their technological future because these films are supposed to "record and mirror the white man's vision of future life." In science fiction movies the white man "has assigned himself centrality and placed people of color at the periphery and margins. (…) In this future world, people of color will have been divested of their cultures and disconnected from their communities."[2] Even *The Matrix,* with its vigorous visions of an Afro-future that remain perhaps unique in the world of science fiction, does not transgress this scheme. Claudia Springer has shown that, though the city of Zion is populated predominantly by black people, the trilogy remains "immersed in the cultural beliefs and film conventions of the 1950s" (2005, p. 59), reinstating James Snead's principle that "[blacks] are being taken out of history into the realm of myth."[3]

The conclusion is that in *The Matrix*, like in any other science fiction movie, the image of black people remains dissociated from a civilized, technology-determined "white" future—which does not mean that black people have no positive role to play. On the contrary, while in *The Matrix* the white (inhuman) administrators make the process of human reproduction more sophisticated in technological terms (until it is no longer human), the black community is destined to guarantee the reproduction of "real" biological bodies. According to Springer, we are here confronted with "a racist paradigm associating black people with authenticity and life and white people with artifice and death" (p. 94). Or, as Lisa Nakamura has put it, in *The Matrix*'s techno-future "blackness is represented as the source of human agency" and race appears as "an essential quality of being 'real', or being 'human', with whiteness occupying the null zone all too often claimed by whites" (Nakamura, 2005, p. 132).[4]

2. The White Negro

Technically speaking, Viagra enhances the human reproduction process; culturally speaking, the drug is not meant to be in the service of reproduction. It becomes clear that any possible script for a Viagra clip, which insinuates the positive value of a technology-invested future in which men can have sex until the last breath without caring about reproduction, faces immense conceptual difficulties when it comes to the incorporation of black people. If blacks were allocated the *Matrix*-role of "human agency" and of the "real biological body," they simply would not *need* Viagra. On the other hand, if they were depicted as marginalized individuals "divested of their cultures and disconnected from their communities," as it usually happens in science fiction films, they would have *no access* to state-of-the-art technology like Viagra.

To this problem there is only one solution: The white man has to integrate into himself those sexual instincts that used to be linked to blackness. With Viagra, the civilized (though occasionally impotence-stricken) white male has made a decisive step not only towards immortality but towards what has for centuries been seen as a typical feature of blackness. Through Viagra the white man has become *virtually* black without embracing black *reality*.

The incorporation of black into white follows the smooth lines of a virtuous and technically controlled program that can be best carried out by surfing on the waves of an age old project: Viagra has to become *cool*. Both Viagra's moral status and its signification as a lifestyle drug depend on the precise meaning of coolness in American society. The problem is that coolness simultaneously represents Viagra's primary *moral* and *cultural* stance. To "be cool" means to assume a moral responsibility and master one's instincts, but it is also through coolness that Viagra manages to become a *cultural icon*. This ambiguity lends Viagra a considerable amount of cultural dynamics because while the drug negates Puritanism—the clips are simply too obscene—Viagra remains compatible with conventional Puritan moral rectitude because any obscenity associated with it exists only in potential (virtual).

The grammar underlying the double status of Viagra (as a simultaneously moral and pop-cultural instance) is relatively easy to explain because there have always coexisted two forms of coolness in America: First there is the white American cool, which is a Republican ideal ascribed to "rational, ascetic, and self-governing individuals" (Takaki, p. ix) able to "repress [their] emotions, to think more clearly and to effect a more 'objective' intellectual analysis" (Dinerstein, 1998, p. 253). According to R.D. Laing, this sort of coolness led to a fragmentization of the self, to "bodies half dead; genitals dissociated from heart; heart severed from head; head dissociated from genitals."[5]

The second notion of coolness, which is most commonly recognized as such outside the US, is of African American origin and has been developed by blacks as a defense mechanism against the degradation of slavery. Because African American cool has been at odds with white Puritan traditions, in the 1950s, some white hipsters began using black cool as a new style of masculinity and as a means of protest against mainstream American society. "The Hipster heralded a new white generation, which believed that purchasing a bit of black earth would lend their lives in Cold War America some badly needed vitality," writes Ian Condry (2006, p. 314). The process of "'blackenizing' America" (White & Cones, 1999, p. 59) began here, but it always worked hand in hand with the white American idea of coolness as an instance of passion control. Somewhere on this trajectory coolness lost its "rebellious status and became the dominant ethic of late consumer capitalism" (Pountain & Robins, 2000, p. 28).

It is important to note that white people never *really* wanted to become black (or what they believed to be black) no matter how hard they tried to be cool. First, as write Majors and Billson, "white males who try to use the cool pose may be perceived by black males as corny" (p. 72). Second, the purpose of the cool culture project had never been to change *reality*. Norman Mailer, in his seminal 1957 essay *The White Negro*, claimed that "hip [or cool] is the affirmation of the barbarian," which never meant that white lifestyles, white cognition, etc. should embrace tendencies of anti-civilization. The correct description of the blackening process of America is rather that whiteness continued to represent the null-zone of racial reality into which "black reality" would be inserted in the form of a *possibility,* as a purely *potential* quality or as a virtual input. If civilization signifies, in the words of Laing, "head dissociated from genitals," virtual blackness enabled whites to maintain a link with male sexuality that functioned through a moment of *potentiality* but has never had any concern in the *real* sexuality of black people.

This is tricky project, which attempts to see "real" blackness in whiteness, has a long tradition in America. These attempts have always been linked to the deepest angers of the national soul. Winthrop Jordan describes in *White over Black* how "Englishmen were attempting to destroy the living image of primitive aggressions which they said was the Negro but was really their own,"[6] and Susan Bordo holds that "since the beginning of the African slave trade, White Europeans have projected *their* anxieties about excess sexuality onto stereotypes of the sexually voracious, over-endowed Black beast" (Bordo, 2002, p. 24).

Black *reality* in white biology and culture needed to be suppressed—though one still desired to be cool. The cool aesthetics of the White Negro could overcome the obstacle only to some extent; we had to wait until the invention of Viagra to find the problem really solved.

Viagra is a little like gangsta rap (the contemporary minstrel show), which "invite[s] the white audience to participate vicariously in a world that [is] both alluring and inaccessible. [In minstrel shows] the stereotypes enacted on stage ripple with sexual potency and license" (Leland, 2005, p. 30). When white people listen to gangsta rap, nothing is real but confined to a play with what *could* happen. In this sense, Viagra represents the latest stage of a blackening process and results in the production of the most recent version of the White Negro. With Viagra, whiteness no longer represents the "soullessness and seeming transparency of modern interface culture" (Nakamura, 2005, p. 132) but is allowed to participate, in the realm of sexuality, in black reality—though only in a virtual fashion.

This explains why in Viagra commercials, the presence of the Black Negro is not wanted: it would remind the White Negro of the *real* sexual body and not merely of it's virtual version. Through Viagra, sexual virility is put to the center of sexual culture, but it resides there not as a real quality but rather *virtually*, in the form of a sexual one-drop rule. Plunging into the commercial world of Viagra, it is easy to recognize how much Viagra imagery is leavened with ideas that seem to flow out of a guide to African American cool culture. The pill is supposed to enable men to overcome puritan dogmas and become virtuous masters of sex. Compare this with a description of a basket ball game: When black people play basketball the game is "improvisatory like black life; formal and yet casual; swift and defiant; held back, contained, and then exploding; full of leaps and breakaway fluid spirits."[7] Black cool itself is described as a "creative, exuberant, Dionysian sensibility wholly at odds with all forms of Puritanism" (Pountain & Robins, 2000, p. 45). This is exactly how Viagra sex is supposed to be like. Viagra is an Afro-disiac.

The problem is that in the cultural imaginary of the nation, white people do not seem to be able to do this naturally. They need Viagra. The popular reasoning seems to be: "There is a black way of playing basketball so there must be a black way of having sex." The anthropologist Thomas Kochman points out that in America "the white mode—that of the middle-class—is relatively low-keyed: dispassionate, impersonal, and non-challenging" (Kochman, 1981, p. 18). In a group discussion that he reports "one black woman, becoming impatient with the wall of white silence, finally said that she thought white men 'couldn't handle it sexually'" (p. 22).

3. Coolness or Machismo?

Black men simply handle it better but can Viagra really help the white man to integrate all those Dionysian and improvisatory qualities into his sex-life? Already Kochman insisted that "white culture develops controls to contain emotions, but few or no controls to manage them at more intense levels of expression" (p. 114). Coolness is the fluidity created by the capacity to hold back and then explode; it is a paradoxical fusion of desire and the mastery of this desire.

How do men use Viagra? Given the evaluations of Viagra as a socio-cultural phenomenon effectuated by sociologists, there are reasons to believe that the use of the drug will lead to classical macho behavior rather than to African American coolness. It all starts with the idea of masculine sexuality, intrinsic to the concept of Viagra, as a force "predominantly portrayed as ever-ready, always willing and desirous, powered by surging hormones and uncontrollable urges."[8] The quick-fix metaphors that consistently neglect the topical (erotic) aspects of sexual activity led an interviewed woman whose partner takes Viagra to comment that "[he seems to think] I've taken the pill; we've got about an hour, I expect you in that time to be acquiescent" (Potts et al., 2003, p. 702). Research by Potts et al. has shown that women claim "sex incorporating Viagra [to be] more likely to involve less time spent on pleasurable activities other than penetrative sex" (ibid.) and a man using Viagra reports that he "could be completely uninvolved emotionally and yet still have a rock hard erection" (Potts et al., 2004, p. 496).

Of course, all this is *not* very cool but comes closer to a caricatured image of machismo. Even more, the entire Viagra project lets the white man appear in a grotesque way as a twenty-first century re-edition of the stereotypical black man from the time of slavery. In this manner, Viagra reduces men, just like the Negro in Frantz Fanon's famous analysis, to a penis: "One is no longer aware of the Negro, but only of a penis: The Negro is eclipsed."[9] Viagra, which is marketed as an enrichment of masculinity represents rather its impoverishment because the Viagra machine, instead of fostering coolness, merely highlights the "compulsive masculine alternative" of coolness, which is, according to Majors and Billson, *machismo* (1992, p. 34). When Majors and Billson provide a definition of machismo it sounds indeed as if they were talking about Viagra: "In compulsive masculinity, typical masculine values become a rigid prescription for sexual promiscuity, manipulation, thrill-seeking (…) violence. Cool is not macho" (ibid.). It has been said that Viagra is "dedicated to the revitalization of a 'true manhood' emasculated by feminism" (Traister, 2000, p. 278). Machismo is another word for the simplistic denial of puritan conventions that remain only barely disguised by a civilizational rhetoric.

4. Viagra and Race

It is ironical that Viagra appears just at the moment when we were beginning to doubt that race really exists. Today, most enlightened people have accepted the fact that race is not "real" in the sense of an unquestionable biological fact, but rather socially constructed. Anthony K. Appiah and Naomi Zack have convincingly shown that the existence of race cannot be scientifically proven explaining that "it is hard to classify people objectively into small sets of populations; and whichever way you do it, it will turn out that, for biological purposes, your classification will contain almost as much human genetic variation as there is in the whole species" (Appiah, 1996, p. 69).[10] Also Zack insists that "the ordinary concept of race in the United States has no scientific foundation. Yet rational people still retain this concept" (1993, p. 18). Philosophers are apparently ahead of the movement because Donna-Dale Macano affirms "that race as a social construct is, by now, old news, at least in philosophical circles" (2003, p. 214).

The problem is that the concept of race *does* constitute a reality since even "rational people" will hold that a person *is* black and not that s/he is "white though submitted to the concept of blackness." Are Appiah and Zack not running in open doors because a large part of the biological concept of race has always been established *through culture*? Stow Persons for example, holds that "the primary and distinctive feature of racism was identification of biological race with culture. It identified a race as a group of people having unique cultural characteristics and playing a unique role in history" (Persons, 1975, p. 297).

Race might be "only" a phenomenon of social construction, but it is nonetheless real. Is it? There are situations where pseudo-scientific facts and social constructions are so much intermingled that a "reality" seems to produce itself out of itself, being neither scientific nor socially justified. The famous case of the Creole gentleman Homer Adolph Plessy whom the Supreme Court of the United States, though he obviously "looked white," disallowed in 1896 to ride the white railroad car, shows the paradoxical conditions of the *being* of race in the United States. Plessy "could certainly have passed in most places for white [but] discovered (…) that the supreme Court of the US proposed to treat him as a Negro" (Appiah, 1996, p. 77). For Appiah, "Plessy vs. Fergusson reflected the extent to which the Louisiana Purchase effectively brought even that state gradually into the American mainstream of racial classification" (ibid.) and this classification is "reality" until today. Still in 1986, a woman who looked white was declared to be 3/32 parts black and therefore submitted to the concept of blackness (J. Davis, 1995, p. 105). The one-drop rule (hypodescent)[11] applies in Mississippi where it equals 1/64 black and in Louisiana where it equals 1/32 black (Hershel, 1995, p. 175).

What does this say about racial "reality"? Was Plessy, as Stephen Satris puts it, "really" black (Satris, 1995, p. 59) because of a "really" black ancestor? In that case, "black reality" has been transformed into a *concept* that claims to be real, even when the phenomenal reality looks otherwise. Scientifically speaking, the "one drop" rule is irrelevant to the formation of race but can get empowered within a social game that interprets "the drop" as *potentially* or *virtually* powerful or, as it happened in US history, as *virtually* threatening.

Obviously, "the drop" is the precursor of the gene as it exists in another compartment of today's contemporary popular imaginary. Just like the gene, the "one-drop" does not exist in a real and actual form but is only *made real* and actual in the same way in which a presumably virtual sex drive is made *actual* through Viagra. In any scientific or socially supported equation, the gene is as useless as the "drop." What matters is not really the drop but the *potency* or the *virtual power* of the drop. Thomas Shannon explains that

> anthropometric characteristics, including skin color, demonstrate the selective effects of different climates to which modern humans have been exposed in the course of their migrations over the Earth's surface. They vary especially with latitude. By contrast, genes are considerably more useful as markers of human evolutionary history, especially migrations. They vary more with longitude. (Shannon, 2005, p. 278)

The racial reality of the one-drop rule is self-sufficient and grounded by establishing a circular connection between the "scientific" and the cultural. Society rarely permits cultural realities to *entirely* flow out of that culture's standards, but often attempts to scientifically justify its perception of reality. Something like this happened with the one-drop rule and today it happens with Viagra: a "scientific" concept that has no meaning outside the *culturally* determined realm within which it appears is used as an instance of determination supposed to function also *outside* its original context where it exists *only* as a potentiality.

Within any one-drop imaginary, racial reality, though being invisible, lingers on the ground of existence and can become manifest at any moment. This happens for example, in the 1931 play *Brass Ankle* by Du Bose Heyward, in which a "black" woman who passes for white "bore a 'throwback' child who revealed her mixed African, Native American, and Caucasian racial heritage" (Giles, 1995, p. 67). The black child "proves" that racial reality, as a subterranean virtual genetic power, even where the "real" component is smaller than those of quadroons or octoroons, *can* become concrete and real. The significance of "race as a cultural construct" is that of race as a potential/virtual quality, which permits the illicit scientification of a non-scientific concept.

5. Virtual Race

Etymologically, virtual comes from the Latin *virtus* (strength, manliness, virtue) in the sense of the potential, which is in the power (virtus) of the force.

Aristotle distinguishes between the virtual and the actual, holding that the oak is *virtually* present in the acorn. "The virtual is not that which is deprived of existence but that which possesses the potential, or force, of developing into actual existence," says Ryan. It is therefore useless to say, as Appiah seems to do with the help of Ian Hacking,[12] that race is only a label and that this label claims to be more real than the physical reality perceived. It is meaningless to pretend that race is "only" a cultural construct as long as the concept refers to a virtual scientific quality (a drop of blood or "a handful of genes") that is *potentially* real. Even if race is not scientifically "real" it still is, as also Zack points out, "the result of complex myths and social fictions that form a powerful cultural reality" (Zack, 1997, p. 100). Finally, the concept of "white race" is even more virtual because it bases itself not even on one drop but on the *absence of the very drop*, an idea that we find in Zack's formulation of the white race as a place where "a nothingness" provides that person's identity (Zack, 1993, p. 27).

Above I referred to racial imaginaries suggesting that "the black can be in the white." These imaginaries are diverse, but always contain a virtual moment. The "one drop"—though inexistent in scientific terms—was claimed to be potentially able to change a person from white to black. Winthrop Jordan's example mentioned above, about Englishmen destroying the living image of primitive aggressions represents a variation of this socio-psychological pattern. Jordan claimed that this barbarism is not the Negro's but their own. Being afraid of their own sexual inappropriateness, white people incorporated the *potential* crimes into the black other therefore contributing to the social construction of blackness. This is how Winthrop Jordan continues his description of "black over white":

> We, therefore, do not destroy; it is someone else. We are not great black bucks of the fields. But a buck *is* loose, his great horns menacing to gore into us with life and destruction. Chain him, either chain him or expel his black shape from our midst, before we realize that he is ourselves.[13]

The possible black drop in the white man is potentially dangerous: "If the gates fell, so did humanness; they could not fall; indeed there could be no possibility of their falling, else man was not man and his civilization not civilized" (ibid.). The question is: can the gates fall today when the white man has Viagra? Well, they will not fall because Viagra *is* civilization, it *is* technology, and it is a purely white product.

6. Conclusion

It has been said above that the virtual gene of blackness "defines people as intrinsically threatening and dangerous to white families" (Zack, 1993, p. 27).

Since the invention of Viagra we notice a remarkable parallel between sex and race: everything that has been said in this article about race and its virtual input is also true about sex at the moment it becomes viagrified,[14] that is, at the moment it becomes a matter of a potential (virtual) reality.

A Viagra user "explained that while he no longer found his wife sexually attractive, with the help of Viagra he was able to 'endure' sex with her." We can conclude that this is very far removed from the original idea of coolness as "a paradoxical fusion of desire and the mastery of this desire" discussed above. The virtuous and fluid handling of desire including "the capacity to hold back and then explode" is only possible in a *real* erotic place. Cool sexuality—if that has ever been the project of Viagra sex—would also "include sexual feelings produced without physical touching" (Potts, 2004a, p. 32) and should not be confined to the organic.

Viagra sex is soulless sex, it is binary (phallic/non-phallic) sex that echoes in its simple-mindedness the American parallel of black/white racial binarism based on the one-drop rule. It is the sex of Agent Smith that occupies a white null zone of racelessness as well as of sexlessness in *The Matrix*. The parallels between Viagra sex and racial schemes persist. To de-viagrify and de-virtualize sex means to put it back into a concrete topical context. A similar de-viagrification of race will be carried out at the moment we decide to see race not as a pseudo-scientific, virtual phenomenon but as a spiritual and cultural *reality*. The racial reality of white Americans is, for example, as writes Stow Persons, that "to the original English had been added Dutch, Scandinavian, Scotch-Irish, German, Huguenot, and Celtic-Irish elements. Again, these were kindred races, and the greatness of the American republic testified to the happy combination of qualities emerged from their union" (Persons, 1975, p. 306). That's all there is: no one-drop rule, no potentially threatening powers, no "viagrification."

W.E.B. Du Bois's writings on race confirm this posture. For Du Bois, the most prominent suggestion about race has been to recognize race as a reality that can be complex but that is not supposed to veer off into threatening potentially dangerous realms. Du Bois was convinced that

> one needs to invoke the "subtle forces" of history, law, habits of thought, the end of human striving and religion to account for the distinctive spiritual lives of racial groups. In other words, explaining the unique spiritual message of a race is a matter of the human sciences (history and sociology) not the natural sciences (biology and chemistry). (Blight & Gooding-Williams, 1997, p. 9)

Here race is presented as a socio-cultural reality that is real in the sense of a dramatic flow of "fluid and hybrid identities" and which has made America a *tragic*—and not a *virtual*—land. Racial—as much as sexual—reality is composed of multiple in-betweens, ambiguities, and compositions that no "virtual potency" should try to modify. Racial and sexual realities are not artificial realities of a virtual desire, but erotic realities able to create real desire.

Notes

1. According to Potts (2004) Viagra leads to a confusion of "the boundaries between human and non-human" and to an "amalgamation of the organic and the synthetic" (p. 1).
2. Omolade, 203 (quoted from Helford, p. 3).
3. Snead from Springer 2005, p. 93.
4. Apart from that, Nakamura interprets the coordination of black and white elements in a much less antagonistic fashion than Springer when claiming that *The Matrix* "seems to break new ground in depicting black men in relation to computers" (p. 126).
5. R. D. Laing: *The Politics of Experience* (New York: Pantheon, 1971), p. 55, quoted from Takaki 1979, p. 10.
6. Winthrop Jordan: *White Over Black: American Attitudes Toward the Negro 1550-1812* (Chapel Hill: University of North Caroline Press, 1968), 579, quoted from Takaki, p. 12.
7. Michael Novak, *The Joy of Sports/End Zones, Bases, Baskets, Balls, and the Consecration of the American Spirit* (NY Basic Books, 1976), p. 105 quoted from Caponi, p. 2.
8. J. M. Ussher, *Fantasies of Femininity: Reframing the Boundaries of Sex* (London: Penguin 1997), quoted from Potts 2004a, p. 24.
9. Fanon thought it to be necessary to let this follow by a scientific comment by Dr Pales who confirms that the "average length of the penis among black men of Africa rarely exceeds 120 millimeters (4.6244 inches)" and that Dr. Testut, in his *Traité d'anatomie humaine*, found the same length for white men (ibid.).
10. See also Appiah 1985, p. 35: "The truth is that there are no races: there is nothing in the world that can do all we ask 'race' to do for us."
11. According Reginald Daniel, the rule of hypodescent "emerged in the late 17th and eighteenth centuries as a means of increasing the number of slaves" (Daniel 1996, p. 122).
12. Ian Hacking: "Making up People" in Thomas Heller (ed.), *Reconstructing Individualism: Autonomy, Individuality and the Self in Western Thought* (1986), p. 87: "numerous kinds of human beings and human acts come into being hand in hand with our invention of the categories labeling them." Quoted from Appiah & Gutmann 1996, p. 78.
13. Jordan, 579 from Takaki, p. 12.
14. On the term 'Viagrification' see Glovka et al. 1999, p. 92: "Process to make something excited or stimulated. (…) Everywhere you turn the Viagrification of America proceeds apace."

Twelve

DAVID HUME MEETS VIAGRA: THE MISUSE OF THE SCIENCE OF ERECTILE DYSFUNCTION

Herbert Roseman

1. Introduction

The introduction of Viagra at the close of the twentieth century had a revolutionary impact on both social and sexual norms. Lost in the media publicity and late-night comedian jokes were two revolutions in the science of male impotence. First, this science was transformed from the soft science of psychoanalysis to the hard science of biochemistry, culminating in the creation of Viagra. Driven by the enormous commercial potential of Viagra, the science was retransformed, extending its scope to encompass the well-being of the male, his partner and his family.

The process of scientific revolutions has been modeled by Thomas Kuhn in his book *The Structure of Scientific Revolutions,* arguably the most influential text in the philosophy of science. The most controversial feature of Kuhn's thesis is that, contrary to usual assumptions, revolutions in scientific paradigms ultimately result from the subjective psychological and social preferences of scientists and not from scientific objectivity and rationality. This paper argues that researchers' financial preferences drove both revolutions in the science of male impotence. The commercial value of Viagra and its competitor pharmaceuticals amounts to billions of dollars; consequently, the industry invested heavily in the research that established and enhanced the market for these pharmaceuticals. The investment successfully advanced the science of male impotence, but the success came at a cost to the scientific integrity of the researchers.

This paper begins by summarizing the history of the science of impotence in the light of Kuhn's model. Using historical evidence Kuhn argues that scientific revolutions occur when a new paradigm replaces an old one. However, in the case of the science of impotence paradigm replacement occurred only for the first revolution, the move from the psychological to the biochemical paradigm. In the second revolution, contrary to Kuhn's model, the biochemical paradigm absorbed a new social paradigm, which added the study of impotence's effect on Quality of Life (QOL)[1]. Significantly, the term male impotence was changed to Erectile Dysfunction (ED). The second section of the paper argues that since QOL is a proxy for well-being, the absorbed paradigm moved the science of ED into the normative realm and *inter alia* created an ethically questionable justification for using pharmaceuticals such as Viagra to relieve ED.

The introduction of QOL into the hard science of biochemistry motivated research to relate ED to QOL quantitatively, which necessitated the development of numeric measures of ED. Researchers responded by creating ED indices. The justification for clinical use of these indices on the male population is induction from the statistical results of a sample of men. Induction from a statistical sample is well justified for measures such as height, weight, blood pressure, etc., but there are additional problems in extending induction to created facts, especially when the facts affect the interests of the sponsors of the research. The next section discusses these problems and argues that indices serve the interests of the pharmaceutical companies rather than the interests of the patients'.

2. History of the Science of Erectile Dysfunction

In the *Structure of Scientific Revolutions* Thomas Kuhn argues that historical evidence shows science usually progresses in a cumulative fashion but undergoes occasional major paradigm shifts. For Kuhn, there are three stages in the development of a science. First, there is a "pre-paradigm stage" (phrases in quotations in this paragraph are Kuhn's) in which scientists collect facts and theorize on a family of related problems until a paradigm eventually emerges. Second, in Kuhn's next stage, "normal science," scientists engage in "puzzle solving" in an attempt to enhance and expand the central paradigm. If the activities during normal science generate sufficient anomalies, the science reaches a "crisis," and a new paradigm is proposed. The science then enters the third stage, "revolutionary science," in which the old and new paradigms contend, and a victorious paradigm emerges. One of the most controversial aspects of Kuhn's model is that the success of the winning paradigm is based not solely on reason and evidence but also on the personal, political and social preferences of the contending scientists.

Prior to the early 1980's, treatment of male impotence was the purview of the psychiatric profession; impotence was thought to be a phenomenon involving the subject and the psychopathology of his sexuality. In Kuhnian terms the psychological explanation of male impotence could be considered the pre-paradigm phase. In the early 1980's the science of impotence entered Kuhn's 'normal' phase with researchers 'solving problems' in both the psychological and physiological causality of male impotence. In 1983, Dr. Giles Brindley's dramatic demonstration of the injection of a drug to treat impotence was an important anomaly that helped to trigger a new paradigm which competed with the psychological paradigm. Impotence was "all hydraulics" (quoted in Loe, 2004, p. 39) and could be explained physiologically and could be treated mechanically or biochemically by urologists. Because (1) the pharmaceutical companies were heavily financing research in a medical approach to impotence and (2) there was a greater likelihood of insurance paying for medical rather than psychological treatments, the psychological paradigm had no chance to prevail. The percentage of research articles that mentioned psychological factors shrunk from one-half to less than one-fifth (ibid., p. 32). The main body of impotence research moved from analysis of a patient's states of mind to studies of the biology, chemistry and physics of erections, which, for brevity, will be called the 'biochemical paradigm.' Researchers in urological surgery developed a penile implant, which was the most widely used treatment for impotence in the 1980's. A pharmaceutical to treat impotence was also discovered, but unfortunately it had to be injected into the penis immediately prior to intercourse.

The move to the biochemical paradigm set the stage for the serendipitous discovery of the effects of sildenafil, the pharmaceutical whose commercial name is Viagra. Developed as a treatment for angina, sildenafil had the side effect of causing and sustaining erections. After the discovery of Viagra problem solving in the normal phase of the biochemical paradigm concentrated on the physiological and medical research necessary to bring Viagra and competing pharmaceuticals to market.

Pfizer, the company that developed sildenafil, and its competitors recognized the enormous commercial potential of this pharmaceutical. In 2009 the sales of Viagra were about $1.9 billion, and the sales of its major competitors, Cialis and Levitra (developed by Eli Lilly and Bayer) were $1.6 and $0.4 billion for a total market of almost $4 billion. Since the direct cost of a pharmaceutical is only about 15 percent of its selling price, these products have a significant effect on the profitability of their corporations. The competition between these products is intense, with the sales growth rate of Cialis and Levitra far exceeding that of Viagra.[2]

The enormous economic potential of these pharmaceuticals eventually resulted in the second major paradigm shift in the science of impotence: the extension of the science to QOL. The first move towards this paradigm, whose significance may not have been perceived by researchers, was a change in the language used to designate 'impotence' to erectile dysfunction[3] (ED). In 1993 the National Institute of Health (NIH) Consensus Development Panel on Impotence gave its imprimatur to ED, defining it as "the inability to achieve or maintain an erection sufficient for satisfactory sexual performance." This change in language was more significant than mere terminology. The term ED suppresses the highly negative connotation of 'impotence' with an acronym which is more clinical and converts 'impotence' from a socially opprobrious psychological problem to a more socially acceptable medical condition such as kidney or liver dysfunction.

Potential users of Viagra could view themselves as addressing a disease rather than a psychological failure. Pfizer's advertising for Viagra featured Vice Presidential candidate Bob Dole encouraging men with ED to seek help from a physician as opposed to a psychiatrist. Perhaps more significantly, 'dysfunction' is a term that is also used for a problem in the functioning of a system: an individual or a social group. ED could be transformed into a problem that affected the well-being of an individual or his QOL. Since the individual is the member of a social group, by extension ED also affects the QOL of the people close to him. To experience ED was to introduce dysfunction into the families and close associates of the sufferer. It became a moral obligation for a patient to eliminate his ED. Moreover, QOL assessment in ED should always include items about the patient's partner and their relationship, because ED is essentially the couple's problem (Althof, 1999, p. 809).

The removal of the stigma of revealing and treating the condition helped to expand the already enormous commercial potential: the market for pharmaceuticals to treat ED has grown at a rate of almost 12 percent per year since 2005, seven years after Viagra's debut. The commercial potential of these pharmaceuticals also triggered a marked increase in ED research, as demonstrated by the significant growth in the number of ED research publications shown in Table 1. As documented in Chapter 2 of Meika Loe's, *The Rise of Viagra,* the pharmaceutical companies financed a significant portion of the research on ED.[4]

Table 1- Number of Journals, Books and Reference Works Published Which Reference ED and QOL

Years	ED Publications	ED and QOL Publications (number)	ED and QOL Publications (per cent)
2005-2009	6,933	2,836	41
2000-2004	3,058	1,187	39
1995-1999	1,367	368	27
≤ 1994	807	155	19
Total	12,165	4,546	37

Source: Science Direct. Searches on 'Erectile Dysfunction' and 'Erectile Dysfunction' *and* 'Quality of Life'

This change in the popular conception of impotence from a shameful psychological condition to a medical condition whose relief was important for the QOL of the patient and others in turn changed the marketing strategy for these pharmaceuticals. Advertising depicted social situations in which the happiness of a man's life, partner and other associates were all positively affected by these pharmaceuticals. The change also motivated the pharmaceutical companies to trigger the second paradigm shift in the science of what was now termed ED: the expansion of the science to the QOL of the patient and his sexual partner, family and close associates. Table 1 demonstrates the significant growth in the percentage of research articles on both ED *and* QOL. ED science remained concerned with the physiological aspects of ED and expanded to the social realm. It now combined the methodologies of the social sciences with those of the biochemical paradigm.

Kuhn's model of theory change cannot account for the second revolution in the science of impotence. He argues that a revolutionary scientific paradigm eventually replaces the old paradigm. For example, the phlogistic scientists' theories of the chemistry of heating metals in the atmosphere were relegated to brief historical mentions by Lavoisier's discovery of oxygen. The revolution in ED science left two interacting paradigms in place: the biochemical sciences of ED and the social sciences that relate ED to QOL. On the other hand, Kuhn's important observation that revolutions in science are dependent upon the subjective perspectives of scientists is useful to understand these paradigm shifts. The financial power of the pharmaceutical companies, which funds much of the research in ED has been the most important factor in the development of the science of ED. Scientists working in the field, who have the "power to choose between paradigms" (Kuhn, 1996, p. 167) and whose livelihood and professional lives are financed by pharmaceutical companies, instantiate Kuhn's observation. They are motivated by the financial power of the pharmaceutical companies.

The ontology of the facts of the two types of sciences that comprise the current paradigm is distinct. John Searle's classification of facts as "brute facts" or "institutional facts" is useful in understanding this distinction. In this context, brute facts correspond to those medical, biochemical and physiological facts which tend to be independent of human opinions. Such facts exist whether or not they are discovered by humans. On the other hand, institutionally created facts, such as those involving ED and QOL, require human institutions for their existence. This distinction in the ontology of brute versus institutional facts should have an important influence on how we philosophically evaluate the science of ED and its effects on QOL. As demonstrated later in this essay, researchers in this area seem insufficiently aware of the force of this distinction.

Scientific research on brute facts uses the methodologies for measuring and analyzing laboratory measurements and physical effects on subjects. Researchers may disagree upon these facts, but theoretically contrary facts can be resolved objectively by performing further measurements. Institutional facts can be the creations of researchers and are subject to the biases of their creators. Scientists often attempt to remove these biases, but the methodologies for removal may also be biased. Most significantly, further measurement of created facts may not resolve discrepancies. The general epistemic values of the scientific enterprise such as accuracy, consistency, and simplicity are more easily realized in sciences dealing with brute rather than institutional facts. In spite of this additional difficulty, practitioners in research on the latter, as scientists, are also often motivated by these values.

A further complication in this context is that QOL is implicitly normative: we all agree that we ought to attempt to achieve a 'good' QOL for ourselves and others. Whether the scientists like it or not, when they attempt to define QOL, they are specifying what is 'good' and prescribing what we ought to do. This is an apt instance of David Hume's observation: "(…) when of a sudden I am surprised to find, that instead of the usual copulations of the propositions *is* and *is not*, I meet no proposition that is not connected with an *ought* or *ought not*" (Hume, 2005 [1739,1740], p. 363). To find a specific, psychometrically sound and relatively uncontroversial measure of an essentially normative concept like QOL seems hopeless, but ignoring this fact suits the purposes of the pharmaceutical companies.

3. Quality of Life, Erectile Dysfunction and Moral Obligation

A. What is Quality of Life as it Relates to ED?

QOL is a term that is used differently in several contexts. In international affairs, countries and regions often evaluate their QOL, which might include measures of educational opportunities, transportation, recreational facilities, degree of pollution in addition to standard of living. For law enforcement QOL is conceived negatively. QOL crimes are acts that create disorder such as graffiti, and vandalism, and acts that result from social decay such as prostitution and panhandling. Similarly, in medicine the idea of QOL is often used negatively. QOL care is administered to a patient and her family when medical treatment stops working in life-threatening situations.

Researchers that relate QOL to ED conceive of QOL as what is generally non-instrumentally good for the life of a person and agree that ED affects QOL negatively. It is difficult to characterize QOL precisely. Table 2 below illustrates an attempt by two ED researchers to formulate QOL. Assuming both authors examined Jones and determined his QOL to their satisfaction, the authors would have created different institutional facts: 'Jones has a QOL equal to QOL_{Althof} ' and 'Jones has a QOL equal to QOL_{Sand}'. It is clear that QOL_{Althof} is radically different from QOL_{Sand}. It is even possible that the two facts 'Jones has a positive QOL_{Althof}', and 'Jones has a negative QOL_{Sand}' could both be true simultaneously.

Table 2- Comparison of Constructs of QOL

Althof	Sand, *et. al.*
Physical functioning	Being in good health
Cognitive functioning	Harmonious family life
Institutional functioning	Good relationship with partner/wife
Global health perceptions	Enjoying life to the fullest
Mood	Satisfying work life or career
Pain	Having a nice home
Vitality	Satisfying sex life
Overall life satisfaction	

Source: Althof (2002, p. 804) and Sand, et al. (2008, p. 589)

There are conceptual problems with both formulations: the items on both lists overlap. For example, for Althof the item 'institutional function' in its usual sense is dependent upon both items 'physical functioning' and 'cognitive functioning', while for Sand 'Enjoying life to the fullest' is dependent upon all other items in the list. As a result of the overlaps and because neither author can claim that his list is collectively exhaustive, neither list of items could be combined to produce a single measure of QOL. As will be seen later one of the objectives of researchers in ED is to develop a specific, psychometrically sound, widely accepted instrument for measuring QOL for patients with ED. Furthermore, since QOL is an essentially normative concept it is difficult to see how it is possible to achieve this objective or whether QOL_{Sand} or QOL_{Althof} better achieves this objective.

4. QOL and Morality

Although QOL *per se* has not been a subject of philosophical discussion, the idea of well-being, what is ultimately good for a person, has been discussed extensively by philosophers, and QOL can be considered a proxy for well-being in this context. Philosophical conceptions of well-being such as "how well a person's life is going for that person" (Crisp, 2009, p. 2) are closely related to the most global components of QOL of both authors, "overall life satisfaction" or "enjoying life to the fullest." Since the pharmaceutical solution to ED improves one's QOL, it can be considered an obligation of act utilitarianism: one's actions *ought* to maximize one's well-being or its equivalent, QOL. Moreover, relating relief of ED to improved QOL solves a problem in utilitarianism recognized by J.S. Mill.

The form of utilitarianism that seems most applicable to moral justification for prescribing Viagra is prudential hedonism, meaning that well-being consists in maximization of the intensity and duration of an individual's pleasure and minimization of the intensity and duration of her pain. But it is difficult to conceive of a successful marketing campaign for Viagra that classifies its users as hedonists. Along with Viagra's marketing strategists, Mill had significant reservations about hedonism. In his essay, *Utilitarianism*, he asserts that prudential hedonism appears to some "as a doctrine worthy only of swine" (Mill, 1998 [1863], p. 55) Mill's response to this problem was to add the dimension of quality to the degree of pleasure; one pleasure can be more valuable than another if those who have experienced both prefer one to the other. Presumably, the pleasure from an evening of attending *Hamlet* is a higher quality pleasure than tossing darts in a pub.

Mill's problem is especially trenchant in the case of Viagra and ED: after all, the direct effect of Viagra is enabling the patient to achieve orgasm. It seems clear that in the spirit of Mill's formulation of utilitarianism, achieving orgasm is closer to tossing darts than to watching *Hamlet.* If the relief of ED is related to an improved QOL, there is logical room to elevate the pleasure that Viagra creates for its user to a higher quality. This higher quality pleasure encompasses the concomitant improvement of the QOL of the patient's close relationships. These components of QOL are indicated by such items as 'harmonious family life' or 'institutional functioning' in Table 2 above. Viagra users will no longer be hedonists proper because their pleasure cannot be determined solely by the intensity and duration of their own sensual pleasure but also includes the well-being of others. Seeking medical help for ED becomes a "responsible act undertaken by respected, honorable men who feel empowered to take their health in their own hands for the sake of their families and their relationships with their partners" (Sand, et. al., 2008, p. 592). Relief of ED by taking Viagra is transformed into higher quality pleasure.

While this facile argument may be sufficient to justify a marketing campaign, it does not stand up to philosophic scrutiny. To analyze the argument first we need to refine the idea of pleasure. There are two sources of pleasure: (1) the sensation of the sexual act for the Viagra user and his partner and (2) satisfaction for himself and others from improvement in such components of QOL as 'harmonious family life.' While Viagra directly advances the former, depending on circumstances, it may or may not advance the latter. In fact, achievement of the former pleasure may be inimical to the latter. For example, Viagra could enable sexual relationships outside of a marriage resulting in disharmony within the marriage or it could promote unwanted sexual demands on a partner. Further, since QOL is a complex measure with several components, more frequent sexual relations may be inconsequential to the QOL of the user and his close relations. All one can conclude is that improved QOL of the user and others may be a side-effect of using Viagra.

The sensual pleasure that results from Viagra is also subject to the paradox of hedonism: like the direct pursuit of happiness, the direct pursuit of QOL may be self-defeating. People who achieve a good QOL are those who successfully involve themselves in activities such as art, religion, sports or study and achieve pleasure as a consequence of these activities. Perhaps the best way to achieve a positive contribution from sexual relations to one's QOL is to concentrate more on the total relationship with one's partner rather than directly pursuing sexual intercourse through medication. If one is experiencing ED, perhaps a better QOL will result by pursuing satisfying sexual relations indirectly by working cooperatively with his partner.

In addition, the idea of QOL as exemplified by Table 2 is an elitist one. The criteria in both tables assume a life in a modern, wealthy and probably Western society. A man living in a ghetto or in an undeveloped nation who is struggling to feed his family would not think the components of either author's QOL would be high priority objectives. Sand's list seems to be directed to a reasonably wealthy homeowner with a family and a career who could be expected to afford Viagra. Finally, if one expects to justify Viagra from a utilitarian standpoint, one must explain why it is ethical to devote the enormous research resources (about 12,000 studies in the last decade) to ED when there are unsolved medical problems such as tuberculosis, malaria, AIDS, etc. whose eradication would generate far greater benefits for a much larger number of humans (see O'Mathúna, this volume, for more on this).

5. Dueling Indices -IIEF versus PAIRS

As shown in Table 1, relating ED to QOL became increasingly prevalent in ED research. Since precise measurement is a widespread scientific value and measures of ED are prerequisite to measuring the effect of ED on QOL, researchers attempted to develop quantitative tools to measure the effect of ED on the relational and emotional domains in addition to the primary sexual domain. Since the former two domains involve social concepts, the methodologies of social science were absorbed into ED research, and researchers began to develop questionnaires to measure ED and QOL.

The first result was a multi-dimensional index called the International Index of Erectile Function (IIEF), which was derived from a self-administered questionnaire. Supported by a grant from Pfizer Inc., the IIEF was created using factor analysis[5] on responses to a 15 item questionnaire. Although some of the IIEF's questions involve the emotional and relational domains, the great majority of its questions are directed to the sexual domain. Not surprisingly, the IIEF demonstrated that patients taking Viagra improved scores on all domains with the greatest improvement in erectile function, while patients given a placebo showed no improvement. Two years later, Pfizer Inc. supported a study (Althof, et al., 1999, p. 803-810) that created more detailed questionnaires, called the Erectile Dysfunction Inventory of Treatment Satisfaction, for both the subject and his partner to assess the outcome of medical treatments for ED on both the subject and on his partner.

Not to be outdone, Eli Lilly and Company, the developer of a competitor to Viagra, Cialis (chemical name tadalafil), funded another study that used factor analysis to develop an alternate index. The marketing campaign for Cialis stresses that its advantage over Viagra is that while Viagra must be taken within four hours of intercourse, Cialis can be taken up to 36 hours prior to intercourse. Cialis users are under less time pressure than Viagra users and can be more spontaneous. This new index, the Psychological and Interpersonal Relationship Scales (PAIRS), was developed from a 23 item questionnaire which stressed questions addressing time concerns and spontaneity. Again not surprisingly, the study demonstrated that assessment of ED treatment should address the time and spontaneity concerns of the subjects and their partners.

The use of both indices in medical practice conforms to standard methodology for statistical measuring tools. The questionnaire results for both studies were related to ED symptoms on a sample of men and were determined to be reliable by various statistical tests. Then, by an appeal to induction, the sample results were deemed valid for any man in the population sampled. For example, any man in the general population whose questionnaire results conformed to a characteristic numerical pattern was deemed to be suffering from ED.

C. D. Broad characterizes induction, which is foundational to the scientific enterprise, as "the glory of science but the scandal of philosophy." Inductive arguments come in many shapes and forms, but all are subject to the unanswerable critique of David Hume, which motivated Broad's remark. Although Hume never uses the term 'induction', he makes it clear that argument is about what we understand as induction. In section IV, Part III of the *Enquiry Concerning Human Understanding* Hume creates a simple but devastating two step proof: (1) "all experimental conclusions [inductions] proceed upon the supposition that the future will be conformable to the past," and (2)" probable arguments [inductive arguments to be discussed here] (…) must be evidentially going in a circle and taking that for granted which is the very point in question" (Hume, 1975 [1777], p. 36).

As opposed to the necessity of deductive arguments, inductive arguments are contingent. The so-called 'problem of induction' is that induction is not a method of proof but is a way of weighing evidence and judging the plausibility of statements. Even good inductive arguments can lead to false conclusions, so one can ask whether any particular inductive argument is reliable. Acceptance of any inductive argument requires satisfaction of two criteria: (1) a sufficient description of the argument and (2) justification of its reliability. (See Lipton for a detailed discussion of description and justification.)

The probabilistic form of the principle of induction is the general form used for the inductions of IIEF and PAIRS (Vickers, 2009, p. 4):

I1. A high proportion p of observed *F's* have also been *G's*
I2. *a*, not yet observed is an *F*
I3. Therefore, it is probable that *a* is a *G*.

For the first criterion of acceptance, sufficient description, the methodology used to develop indices is comprehensively documented in the references. Both studies used factor analysis, a standard statistical technique for reducing a large collection of data to its primary factors that parsimoniously explain the data. (See the Appendix for a brief description of factor analysis.) For example, the Swindle study reduced a data base of thousands of responses to three factors: sexual self-confidence, spontaneity and time concerns.

Justification of the reliability of the induction for the two indices is not as clear. First, factor analysis has a "tarnished reputation" as a scientific tool. (Tabachnik and Fidell, 1981, p. 599). Factor analysis requires subjective judgments in two key steps: (1) factor selection: the trade-off between parsimony of explanation and elimination of statistical error, and (2) the final restatement of the factors. There are no independent statistical criteria to guide these judgments. Second, a more serious problem arises from the use of factor analysis on created institutional facts. Recall Searle's distinction between brute and institutional facts. ED and QOL are not brute facts such as height, weight, age, heart rate, etc. They are created institutional facts such as rankings, preferences, IQ, etc. Standard statistical analyses are reliable for brute facts. One can sample a population for height and infer by induction that the height of an individual in the population will be within a height range with a precisely computed probability. But the induction of the institutional facts raises additional problems, because both *F* and *G* are institutionally constructed, and in this instance *F* is constructed by the researchers themselves.

Hume's argument concerning the circularity of induction pertained to brute facts such as the behavior of billiard balls striking one another, magnetism, explosions, etc. If Hume had thought about it, however, the implications of the extension of induction to institutionally constructed facts would have astonished him. Because institutional facts are created by humans, their existence as facts is dependent on the subject's belief in the fact. Without getting too deeply into the correspondence theory of truth, the reason that we believe snow is white is because it can be objectively verified. The reason we believe facts about currency is because we believe currency was created to have all of the facts that make it currency. This feature of institutional facts makes the circularity involved in inductions concerning institutional facts more vicious than the circularity in inductions concerning brute facts. Moreover, if *F* has been constructed to approximate *G*, the relationship between the two is not causal but one of degree of equivalence. There is further circularity in this kind of induction.

To see this consider the following putative induction:

T1. A high proportion *p* of diners 'tipping 15 percent or more' are 'good tippers.'
T2. Jeff, not yet evaluated, tipped 20 percent.
T3. Therefore it is probable that Jeff is a 'good tipper.'

The first proposition in this induction is a tautology (i.e. $p = 1$), because the fact that a 'good tipper' is one who tips 15 percent or more is an institutionally created fact, which is based upon humans believing in the fact. Therefore, the 'induction' is vacuous. Jeff did not need to use inductive inference to determine his tip. He had the desire to be a good tipper and believed an institutional fact on tipping.

The induction in the context of IIEF and PAIRS is as follows:

E1. A high proportion of men presenting a characteristic pattern on IIEF/PAIRS questionnaires suffer from ED.
E2. Jeff, not yet evaluated, presents this pattern.
E3. Therefore it is probable that Jeff suffers from ED.

The first statement of this induction is not a tautology but a statistical equivalence. For both indices the most statistically significant factors pertain to the NIH definition of ED. Furthermore, it is arguable from both Ockham's Razor and statistical considerations that in both studies only the factor associated with the erectile function domain and one additional factor should comprise the final index. Moreover, the other factors which were included in the final indices should be dropped.[6] The 'characteristic pattern' of E1 would then track the NIH definition of ED even more closely. In short, the statistically significant part of the multi-dimensional scale of both questionnaires essentially corresponds to the NIH definition of ED. Two of the referenced studies (Edwards, D., et al. [2006] and Rubio-Aurioles, et al. [2006]) seem to recognize this and use only the IIEF erectile function domain in their measurements.

There is almost no causal relationship between the indices and ED, and therefore induction is not needed to extend the results to a particular individual. These indices don't relate an underlying psychological or physiological characteristic to a patient's ED; they simply describe him as suffering from ED. The conclusion is that a subject suffers ED from the results of the questionnaires is not an induction but a convention. The questionnaires could be replaced by simply discussing a patient's ED symptoms in some detail. Although it would lack the scientific patina of a statistically calibrated index, a discussion would give the diagnostician a better opportunity to learn something about a patient's circumstances than a self-administered questionnaire would. The questionnaires could be effectively used to structure a conversation about a patient's ED.

Attempting to justify the induction raises additional concerns about the content of the questionnaires. One must assume that the responses to the questions reflect the subject's actual beliefs. Like ED, the process of responding to a questionnaire is a complex psychological interaction with the environment. Questionnaire response may be what the subject believes his responses ought to be, especially when a matter as psychologically charged as the sexuality of the subject is in question. For example, subjects may respond differently depending upon the sex of the administrator. Researchers must also assume that responses to the questionnaire are stable. Responses to such questions as "How likely is it that you will try to end the relationship with your partner during the next year?" (Swindle, et al., p. 24) seem to be extremely vulnerable to instability. The subject may not have thought about the issue raised by the question until he was filling out the questionnaire. If there are cultural stereotypes operating, then the sample results would be highly biased. For example, in the IIEF study (Rosen, et al., p. 830) there is a question that challenges the subject's attitude toward his masculine identity: "How do you rate your confidence [underline is as printed] that you can get and keep an erection?" Such a question is highly susceptible to different cultural constructs of maleness.[7]

Also, these studies appear to be subject to the bias of the researchers. Although the articles for this essay were chosen without considerations of sponsor, all of the research results favored the objectives of the corporation involved in the research. The IIEF study demonstrated that Viagra was more effective in relieving ED than a placebo. As mentioned, the marketing strategy of Eli Lilly, the sponsors of the PAIRS study, stresses the advantage of Cialis over Viagra as related to time and spontaneity. It is a prima facie assumption of folk psychology that sex is usually more enjoyable if there is no time pressure. The marketing strategists for Cialis clearly assume this, as did the questionnaire developers and the respondents to the questionnaire. In the PAIRS study, 18 of the total of 23 questions specifically refer to time or spontaneity. It would be very surprising if a factor analysis of such a questionnaire did not reveal that time and spontaneity were statistically significant. As another example, a study (Rubio-Aurioles, et al. [2006]) sponsored by Bayer, the manufacturer of Levitra demonstrated that significantly more men preferred this pharmaceutical over Viagra.

Although the indices presented in the research appear to be cardinal numbers, they are actually invalid combinations of ordinal numbers. Ordinal numbers can only tell us whether one answer to a question is higher or lower (better or worse) than another, but not the size of the difference between answers. As a simple example, although we can say the horse that finished first in a race performed best, it is impossible to say whether a horse that finished first and fourth in two races performed worse than one who finished second in both races by adding the ordinal numbers that represent the finishes. We need to know finish times, payoffs or some relevant number that can be combined arithmetically (technically, measured on a linear scale). The arithmetic combination of ordinal numbers is valid only if it can be shown that the difference between them is equal. It is difficult to see how this criterion could hold for the ED indices. Both indices use multiple scales which often vary from question to question. For example, in the IIEF study for Questions 1 and 2 the ordinal numbers 2 and 3 represent the answers "A few times" and "Sometimes" while the same ordinal numbers represent the answers "Very Difficult" and "Difficult" for Question 5. The likelihood that the interval between these two sets of ordinal numbers is the same for both questions for all respondents is highly unlikely. It becomes even more unlikely when this restriction is applied to all responses to all questions in the questionnaire. An IIEF erectile function score of 25.8 appears to have the same numeric properties as a measurement of body temperature of 98.6, but the former is theoretically flawed while the latter is an excellent guide. Medical practitioners that use these indices and their patients are, in all likelihood, unaware of this theoretical problem or its ramifications.

Finally, even if we ignore the previous problems, the most important question of how ED relates to QOL requires scrutiny. Having a good QOL is a multi-dimensional construct dependent upon culture and many personal factors such as education, health, job satisfaction, financial security, relationships, etc. Can we seriously believe that QOL will not be strongly affected by non-sexual factors or that ED's impact on QOL is independent of these factors? That is not to argue that ED does not in general affect QOL negatively, but the degree of the relationship is highly situational. Until this relationship is resolved, the utility of a statistically characterized relationship between QOL and ED for any individual male has limited clinical usefulness.

On the other hand, having an index that appears precise and scientifically based is highly useful to the pharmaceutical companies. It allows medical practitioners to justify a prescription by appealing to a number which, on the surface, is as objective as a measurement of blood pressure rather than a detailed and critical clinical analysis of a patient's medical and psychological background. The funding of research that generates these indices indicates that the pharmaceutical companies believe that more drugs will be prescribed.

6. Conclusion

What makes Thomas Kuhn's writings controversial is that he argues that in scientific revolutions scientists are motivated by factors other than scientific objectivity, rationality, and evidence. Most of Kuhn's historical evidence comes from physics and chemistry, sciences that are based upon brute facts. Kuhn's work has little to say about sciences in which the researchers help to create and not to discover the facts of their science. Objectivity is more challenging in such sciences, especially when the livelihood of the researchers is determined by institutions with a significant financial stake in the outcome of the research. In such situations, Kuhn's observation that scientific research is influenced by the preferences of scientists pertains to normal science and to scientific revolutions.

This essay has argued that both the revolutions in the science of impotence and the development of indices to quantify ED, an instance of normal science, have been unduly influenced by the financial power of the pharmaceutical companies. Ironically, the development of the indices was motivated by an important scientific value, precision of measurement. Unfortunately the institutionally created facts, ED and QOL, are too poorly defined to measure precisely. Consequently this essay has also argued that the indices are fatally flawed as a medical tool. The indices are falsely precise numbers, which encourages medical practitioners to prescribe Viagra or its competitor pharmaceuticals without critically evaluating the patient's situation. This argument is debatable, which is characteristic of the learning process that is part of science. What is even more troubling is the support that scientists provided to the pharmaceutical companies actually helped to create invalid ethical criteria that justify the use of these pharmaceuticals for treating ED. These kinds of activities vitiate the values of science and transform scientists into a clever group of business men mainly motivated by money.

Appendix

Factor Analysis

Factor Analysis is a statistical technique that seeks to reduce a large number of variables into subsets of variables that are correlated with one another but not correlated with variables in the other subsets. These groups or subsets are called factors and are meant to reflect parsimoniously the underlying processes that created these variables. For example, suppose a researcher is trying to discover the characteristics of women predictive of satisfaction with their partner's use of Viagra. As a first step the researcher might develop a questionnaire that collects data that researchers believe may be associated with their satisfaction with their partner's use of Viagra from a population of women. The questionnaire might be comprised of questions on age, income, education, personality factors, participation in leisure activities, types of literary interests, attitudes, etc. The next step is to prepare a mathematical representation of the statistical correlation (technically a correlation matrix) of each pair of questionnaire responses. For example we might find that subjects with high incomes are likely to have high educational levels and there is only a small likelihood these subjects will be involved in bowling. Next, the correlation matrix is subjected to a factor analysis program which groups the questionnaire responses that are statistically correlated with one another into factors. In our example factor analysis might find groups of questions related to social class, religious affiliation, political affiliation, athletic involvement, etc.

Since the objective is to reduce the responses to a minimal set of factors, the researcher must then select the factors that will adequately explain the data statistically. The more factors selected the better will be the statistical explanation of the data, but the fewer the number of factors the better will the objective of parsimony be satisfied. The selection of factors to include is a judgment of the researcher. Selection can be controversial and questionable because there is no external independent statistical measure to test the solution. There is only the criterion of interpretability which can, of course, be highly subjective.

Factor analysis computes a variable known as an eigenvalue for each factor that is helpful in making this judgment. There are rules of thumb about eigenvalues to assist this judgment, but there is no requirement to use these rules. A technique that is often used is the screen plot. The eigenvalues are plotted along the x axis from highest to lowest. The accepted factors are the ones associated with the highest eigenvalues that can be grouped around a single straight line. The technique is not exact. It involves a subjective visual judgment of when the first rejected eigenvalue cannot be grouped along the line.

In our example the researcher might decide that economic class and religious affiliation are sufficient to statistically account for the questionnaire responses because factor analysis has shown that the next most statistically significant factor, political affiliation, has a significantly smaller eigenvalue than religious affiliation. On the other hand, if the researcher believes that political affiliation is an explanatory factor he may elect to include it if the eigenvalue is not too low (less than one is a rule of thumb). Presumably, the factors selected are judged to be the best set of explanatory variables for satisfaction with their partner's use of Viagra

After the factors are selected they are submitted to a mathematical analysis that re-computes the factors to improve their interpretability. In other words the mathematical combination of the responses to the questions is varied to better understand the factors. But there is no external criterion for evaluating the literally infinite ways of the re-computation of the factors. The re-computation selected by the analyst is again based on interpretability which can also be controversial. The analyst should not be surprised if results are not replicable.

Factor analysis can have great utility in reducing a large number of variables to a much smaller number of factors that underlie the process that generated the variables. Ironically, the power of the method to perform this function often leads to its misuse: one can usually find affiliation of various items on questionnaires leading one to believe that an underlying pattern has been discovered. In summary, the results of a factor analysis must be interpreted with extreme care:

> ... FA [factor analysis] is frequently used in an attempt to 'save' poorly conceived research. If no other statistical procedure is applicable at least the data can be factor analyzed. Thus in the minds of many, FA is associated with sloppy research. (Tabachnick & Fidell, p. 599)

Notes

1. Warning. There are several acronyms in this essay which may be annoying to the reader. I apologize in advance. These acronyms are the terminology of this science, and I couldn't see how to eliminate them. In fact I left several out.
2. Sales figures were sent to me in a private communication from a research analyst from a financial institution who prefers to remain anonymous. I will forward the report upon request. I calculated the approximate cost of sales figure from Pfizer's 2005 annual report.
3. This definition is only partially helpful because the meaning of 'satisfactory sexual performance' is open-ended. One would ask the questions "Satisfactory to whom?" and over what time period. One could also ask "What is meant by 'sexual performance'?"
4. Although it is beyond the scope of this article to determine precisely the degree of financing of ED research by pharmaceutical companies, it is interesting to note

that *all* of the research references in the bibliography of this article involved scientists from pharmaceutical companies. This evidence can only be considered anecdotal, but pharmaceutical company involvement was not one of my criteria in selecting articles for my research.

5. A brief description of factor analysis is given in the Appendix. Strictly speaking the IIEF was developed using principle components analysis which is very similar to factor analysis. The differences between the two, the way that the variance of the observed variables is analyzed, is irrelevant to these considerations.
6. Statisticians alert. For both studies the eigenvalue for the factor on erectile function was approximately twice as large as the next largest eigenvalue. In the IIEF study the eigenvalues for erectile function, overall satisfaction, orgasmic frequency, sexual desire and intercourse satisfaction were 4.72, 2.22, 2.03, 1.81, and 1.47 respectively. For the PAIRS study the factors sexual self confidence, spontaneity, time concerns were 7.81, 4.17 and 2.10 respectively. I did a scree analysis for both studies. In my opinion the scree analysis shows that for the IIEF study the factors erectile function and overall satisfaction should be included but orgasmic frequency, sexual desire and intercourse satisfaction should be excluded. For the PAIRS study the factors sexual self confidence and spontaneity should be included but time concerns should be excluded. Of course this is open to argument.
7. For example, in the MALES study (Sand, et. al.) of the constructs of maleness, the variation by nationality of the percentage of men reporting that "being in control of your own life" went from 17% in France to 44% in Germany with eight different nationalities sampled.

Thirteen

A SHORT NOTE ON VIAGRA AND THANATOS

Herbert Roseman

The obvious god from Greek Mythology to associate with Viagra is Eros. In this volume Stephanie Bourgault makes this association in her title and Thomas Kapper associates Aristotle's discussion of friendship with Eros. These two authors, and I suppose many others, correctly reason that since Viagra effects sexual relations, it is related to sexual love. But does Viagra have any relationship with Thanatos and death? It may be surprising that Darwinian thinking demonstrates that Viagra may also have an effect on our senescence and death.

To understand the relationship between Viagra and Thanatos it is necessary to have a basic understanding of the biological meaning of fitness and the biological reason for death. For biologists, the meaning of fitness is simply the relative ability of an organism to transmit its genes to the next generation. Darwinian evolution is about fitness. The Darwinian law of evolution can be stated succinctly and causally as: evolution is caused by the differential reproduction (fitness) of elements with variable heritable characteristics. These heritable characteristics are encoded in an organism's genes, which are expressed in what is called the organism's phenotype, i.e. its observable characteristics. Thus, natural selection will favor the transmittal of genes expressed in those variations in phenotypes that cause them to grow and reproduce vigorously. Such phenotypes will enjoy more reproduction of themselves than other organisms. Consequently, after the age when an organism has finished passing on its genes, natural selection does not 'care' about what happens to the phenotype. And as Darwin stated, "any variation, however slight, if it be in any degree profitable (…) will tend to the preservation of that individual, and will generally be inherited by its offspring" (Darwin, 2005, p. 378).

Due to advances in medicine and sanitation, human life expectancy has been rising steadily for the past century or so. In the past decade or so researchers have focused on the biology of aging and found that aging results from what can be thought of as harmful actions by our cells. (All of the biology of aging discussed here and much more is described in language accessible to the layman in Jonathan Weiner's elegantly written book, *Long for the World*.) The human body is comprised of trillions of cells which are miraculously functioning miniature factories. Like processes in all factories, cellular operations have defects that inevitably result in damage that accumulates with time, and at some point the cell can no longer function and dies. If a sufficient number of cells die, then the organism itself dies. Aging is driven by molecular defects in our cells rather than from a genetic program.

Aubrey de Grey, a well known biological theorist, argues that we can feasibly engineer negligible senescence by attacking seven of these defects. De Grey argues that accumulating damage in our cells causes them to "flail about in increasingly, desperate, disorderly panicked attempts to keep their heads above waters of the aging process" (quoted in Weiner 2010, p. 102). The way to achieve essentially unlimited life expectancy is to prevent or clean up the detritus that is the result of cellular functioning and accumulates within and around our cells by pursuing what de Grey terms Strategies for Negligible Senescence (SENS).

The question then becomes why hasn't natural selection adopted such strategies. For example, why hasn't natural selection, which has evolved human organs as complex as the eye, created a mechanism for improving the relatively simple structure and functionality of the lysosome, the organelle in our cells that digests potentially harmful enzymes? Rather, evolution has designed the lysosomes to allow some of these enzymes to accumulate in the cell, damage its operation and result in its eventual death. Sir Peter Medawar, a Nobel Prize winner for immunology, has answered this question. Natural selection is a process that allocates the scarce resources and energy available to an organism for the sole purpose of increasing its fitness. Since the world tended to be a precarious place when humans evolved, natural selection produced organisms that spread their genes when young before they were either killed by a predator, disease or an accident. In such a situation natural selection would cause resources to be allocated mostly for the benefit of the young to aid the process of reproduction. Since genes that produce phenotypes that extend life beyond the years of reproduction have no effect on fitness, the energy expended on prolonging the existence of a body could be better used to increase the ability of the young to reproduce. Prolonging the life of an organism after it has survived beyond the age of reproduction is a disadvantage to natural selection because it wastes resources that could have been devoted to fitness. Therefore, evolution has built aging and death into our phenotypes.

What has this to do with Viagra? Viagra, if used for reproductive sex, increases the fitness of males by increasing the number of opportunities for transmitting its genes to the next generation. Since scientific innovation has greatly reduced the probability of death by disease or accident in many cultures, Viagra has extended the age that males can transmit their genes. Thus, Viagra has increased the fitness of older men. Natural selection now has an "incentive" to extend the lives of males because they can transmit their genes later in life. Moreover, as more of these fortunate males enter the population, there will be more incentive to promulgate the use of Viagra and develop products that improve the functionality of Viagra. The evolution of the increase in longevity and the Viagra culture are said to coevolve; they are linked to one another.

As a hypothetical example of this incentive, consider a man who has a dominant mutation that improves the functionality of the lysosomes in his neurons in his brain which extends his life. Although the man would live longer than other men, before the advent of Viagra this mutation would have no evolutionary effect. The age at which the man had the ability to copulate would be the same as a man who did not have the mutation. But, with Viagra, the man with the favorable mutation will be able to pass this mutation on to offspring for a longer period of time than those who lack this mutation; his fitness will increase compared to the others. Recall that Darwin observed that even a slight increase in fitness in an organism will tend to increase the offspring of that organism versus others of his species. Moreover, when organisms with this mutation become more prevalent in the population the use of Viagra and any further developments that extend the age of reproduction will also increase. This process will feed back on itself producing a population with a greater percentage of humans with this mutation and its phenotype, greater longevity. It is worth noting that this advantage will also accrue to female offspring of the males with the mutation who will in turn pass it along to their offspring.

The Viagra phenomenon presents a unique case in the coevolution of culture and genes. The classic study of such coevolution is presented in *Coevolution, Genes, Culture and Human Diversity*, by William H. Durham which discusses coevolution of lactose absorption and dairying culture. Durham convincingly demonstrates that over many generations humans in societies lacking sufficient exposure to the sun developed both biological mechanisms for lactose absorption and darying cultures. There was a ratchet-like progression; as lactose absorption increased so did the depth and breadth of the darying culture which resulted in the increase in the use of dairy products and ability to absorb lactose.

The biological side of the Viagra/life extension coevolution is more powerful than the darying/lactose absorption. The effect of lactose absorption on fitness is indirect while the effect of longevity on fitness is direct. The improvement in fitness for lactose absorbers is a result of improved health (better calcium absorption, decline in rickets, etc.) so the opportunities to transmit the lactose absorbing gene was subject to many contingencies. Since humans are highly sexually motivated, males with the life-extending mutations will, with the aid of Viagra, have more opportunities over a lifetime to transmit their genes. In addition, the modern communications media and science spread the Viagra culture much more rapidly than, say, the promulgation of bovine myths amongst early occupiers of the Scandinavian countries. Because both the biological and cultural dimensions of the longevity/Viagra coevolution are both stronger than that of the darying/lactose absorption, the former should theoretically occur more rapidly, especially in reproductively isolated human communities.

Of course natural selection is, by its very definition, a slow process. To date, increasing longevity has been the purview of medical science, sanitation, immunology, etc. The inefficient process of natural selection will require many generations to sort out the mutations that increase our life span. Furthermore, if Aubrey de Grey's program for life extension is successfully implemented, its cultural effects will, in all likelihood, swamp natural selection's contribution. Still, as philosophers, we are motivated to discover and analyze all logical possibilities of this new phenomenon. Who would have thought that Viagra may slow down "swift Thanatos" and give future philosophers more time to extend these analyses?

Fourteen

COMPARATIVE MELIORATION AND PATHOLOGICAL PATHOGENIZATION IN VIAGRA MARKETING

Roman Meinhold

1. Introduction

Viagra is everywhere, empty packages can be seen on rural African dirt roads and beside trash cans in the streets of Bangkok. But most often I am confronted with it when emptying my email spam folder. According to the subject lines of Viagra spam messages men are not potent enough. Potency appears in comparatives but often without concrete quantifications. By avoiding quantifications the marketers evade being accusable of exaggerations since quantified comparatives would illogically surpass empirical superlatives. Today's men have the impression that their sexual "performance" must be pathologically suboptimal since a "harder," "bigger," "longer" "tool" and "more powerful" erections and orgasms can always be achieved with certain forms of "lifestyle medication." This paper aims at elucidating a particular aspect of the anthropologic-(pop)cultural relation of man and Viagra: The pathological pathogenization, is a trend to define everything as sick, unhealthy and dysfunctional (pathogenization) with an economic agenda in the backdrop, that is sick, unhealthy, and a dysfunction in itself (pathological). In the first part the paper analyzes the philosophic-anthropological implications of the comparative melioration employed in Viagra and other lifestyle products' marketing. Then I will explain why certain characteristics of the Western medical system invite medical treatment such as that of Viagra. Finally I will elucidate the pathologization as pathological cultural manifestation employed by marketing strategists for economic reasons. The paper concludes with an appeal to redirect intellectual and monetary resources into education for health consciousness and into preventive measures for health.

In order to demonstrate that the comparatives employed in Viagra advertising are pathological and pathogenic I am going to bring a specific anthropological condition in relation to a certain trend in popular culture. This approach follows a particular marketing strategy employed for many popular products and services. The anthropological condition to which I refer—humans' drive to improve conditions and things while having a comparing eye on similar conditions and things (comparative melioration)—is quite frequently employed in marketing strategies (Meinhold, 2005, 2007, 2009). A marketing strategy in its own right is the pathologization, which can also be seen as a trend in popular culture (especially in the beauty-health-lifestyle-sexual performance sector). The two strategies combined—the pathologization on the one hand and comparative melioration on the other hand—seem to be a very powerful strategy to sell insurance and medical services or products. An example of how this is done can be exemplified in the case of Viagra: *"more than half of men over 40 have some difficulty getting and maintaining an erection"* and this is *"a real medical condition"* (pathologization), but in most cases *"harder longer lasting erections"* (comparative melioration) can be achieved by using Viagra (all quotes from the Viagra website). I will deal with the issues of comparative melioration first, and then turn the focus to the pathogenization.

2. Longer, Bigger, Thicker, Harder...
Comparative Melioration, a Philosophic-Anthropological Condition

Man and his being were admittedly always conceived of in the comparative: in art, medicine, ethics and utopia. Melioration (Lat. *melior* 'better', comparative of *bonus* 'good') is the anthropological condition of the human striving for what is *better*, especially for *the better life*. I am here utilizing a concept that—like the term *sustainability*—comes from the sphere of forestry and agriculture, where it refers to the management of naturally sparse resources. Melioration refers to cultural (i.e. humanly devised) measures to improve the quality of the soil. Analogously, humans can be considered as a (nature-given) resource which, like arable land, is not removed from cultural influences but which—unlike arable land—is also able to 'cultivate' itself. The concept of melioration can then be described as the constant striving of humanity for *enhancement* or *improvement* that can be observed since the Palaeolithic Age within all cultural spheres. Already in the Old Stone Age, people sought to improve their surroundings in order to 'live better', whether by using primitive tools or building dwellings. All world religions feature the improvement of virtues. Any artistic activity, regardless of the artistic outcome, results in a melioration of the artist's abilities. The striving for the "more beautiful" and "the better" represents an anthropological constant that not only manifests itself within the typical spheres of the arts, architecture, and design but also in fashion and in medicine. Humans do not only use aesthetic norms outside themselves, in art and architecture, for example, but also use them *on themselves*. Humans consider themselves to be a malleable 'material' that can be improved and augmented. The arrival of gene technology ushers in a new era of removing deficiencies and of self-improvement, i.e. the anthropotechnological melioration of human beings in general. By anthropotechnology (cf. Sloterdijk, 1999) I mean the technology used by human beings to ameliorate their own bodies or those of others; the *homo faber* becomes a *"homo faber fabricatus"* (Rauscher, 2000, p. 17). In an age of biotechnology we are faced with the problem of having the possibility of taking genetic measures to bring about the biological melioration—or assumed melioration—of human beings, that could affect future generations, depending to the nature of the intervention. It is at present not possible to say what the long-term ethical consequences may be.

In advertising of Viagra, human striving for enhancement touches valuable but vulnerable issues: maleness, performance, potency, and virility. Advertising for consumer items, and Viagra is no exception, expands the 'original' totality of the human being for strategic reasons beyond man himself to consumer goods and their *meta-goods*. In previous research in this field I have defined meta-goods in the following way: "Meta-goods are *existential, intellectual, psychological, emotional, social,* and *spiritual values* or *symbols*. They are immaterial 'by products' of products or services. When bought, meta-goods are, apparently transferred (in)to the consumer" (Meinhold, 2007, p. 7).

It is only via the consumer goods and meta-goods that the person depicted in the advertisement becomes a complete human being. Via Viagra the potential—or once virile—man becomes again (and thus, rejuvenated) a potent man. Expressed negatively, without the corresponding consumer goods (e.g. Viagra) the human being, according to the advertisements, remains incomplete (and impotent). Advertising promises to make the incomplete individual a totality. Consumer items are to even out individual personal deficiencies, or complete individuality regarding a particular quality that, along with the consumer item, can be purchased as meta-goods. In the case of Viagra that is a better sex life, increased self-esteem, youth, virility or better sexual functionality in particular, and a better life in general.

This evening out of deficiencies and completion of individuality found in the advertising of consumer items and services often speaks in the comparative mode: more beautiful, more successful, more powerful, younger, the consumer becomes 'better' with the aid of (meta-)goods extolled in the advertising. In the realm of sexual performance improving drugs and other products, it is the *harder, bigger, thicker, and longer* (either, elongation or duration) comparatives that are employed.

Arnold Gehlen justified the special position of man in nature because of his being deficiently "*equipped with organic weapons or organic means of protection*" (Gehlen, 1993, p. 17) such as degenerated instincts and modest sensory capacity. He expressed this deficient anthropological constitution of man by the term *creature of deficiencies* (Mängelwesen), a word taken from Johann Gottfried von Herder. Because of the deficient nature of his constitution, man is obliged "*to alter nature, no matter how it is constituted, in such a way that it is expedient to his life*" (Gehlen, 1993, p. 18). According to Gehlen, the deficient nature of humanity is the foundation of culture. If one thinks of such examples as telescopes, night-vision apparatus, diving rafts, etc., it is obvious that by 'nature' human nature may also be meant. Because of its deficits compared with other living creatures that have specialized within a particular environment, it has to try to change or improve it.

If it comes to ED (erectile disfunction) the deficiency appears or increases with age. While in the beginning of Viagra advertisements elderly—often 'otherwise successful'—men featured the adverts, the age of men shown in more recent ads can be estimated around 40 and upwards. From a demographic point of view the population in many countries is growing older, therefore ED constitutes an "epidemic." I will go into depth of the pathologizating nature of this move of declaring something as a pandemic in the sections on pathologization and pathogenization. But I first want to turn once again to the aspect of the comparatives in human striving and to the supposedly superlative or ideal references of such comparisons.

Although one can only partially accept the hypothesis of Gehlen regarding man as a creature of deficiencies—since human beings can find themselves both at a disadvantage and at an advantage, depending on the basis for comparison—when it comes to a comparison of organs and instincts, it must nevertheless be maintained that humans cannot avoid changing nature, or 'improving' it for their own ends. Man is a being that seeks to improve his environment and himself; a being that meliorates his life. Even so, man does not really strive for the '*good* life' but rather for the '*better* life', for in human life the good has something of a 'half-life' about it. On the one hand, Baudelaire is right when saying that man is always "*striving for the ideal*" (Baudelaire, 1988, p. 38), for man has ideals, such as a Platonic idea, as his targets in mind, which he strives for but in fact never attains. Should he even so attain an 'ideal', which in our 'world as a cave' only represents a *supposed* ideal, the "deficiency ideality" of this ideal will soon be revealed and a '*better* ideal' will emerge that by definition deprives the old ideal of its ideal status. In all his daily exertions, man does not ultimately strive for the superlative, for the 'best', but for the 'better', since the 'best' represents an ideal construction that will have to be revised, optimized or improved on, as more experience is gained. The ideal of 'the best life' is utopian in orientation, something that will never be achieved but that can serve as a point of reference that governs melioration. In practice, however, man basically strives for what is better. What is 'better' is measured comparatively with the state arrived at so far. Little is to be found in daily life that cannot be directly subsumed under melioration. Indirectly, every attitude and action contributes to a melioration of life, which is why the *intention* and *striving* to improve plays a crucial role in advertising in general, not only in Viagra adverts.

So melioration, man's striving for a better life, can be assumed to be an anthropological constant that manifests itself in some form or other in all cultural spheres and in every epoch of history. Georg Simmel described the essence of human life by the concepts "more-life" and "more-than-life," where life constantly thinks of itself and relates to itself in the comparative: life transcends itself, it is

> to be understood as something that constantly transcends the boundary of its own 'beyond' and has its own being in this transcendence (…). Life finds its nature, its process in being more-life and more-than-life, and as such its positive is already its comparative. (Simmel, 1999, p. 234)

The "self-transcendence of life" expresses itself in these two complementary forms: more-life as the generation of the living in the sense of the transcending of one's own life by the generation of new life; and more-than-life, that is, the transcendence of the boundary of individual life at the level of the mind via creative power (Simmel, 1999, p. 229). Life transcends more-life when "we call ourselves creative," Simmel speaks of more-than-life, which is "the nature of mental life itself" (p. 232). Both comparative forms of life together constitute human life as such. The affinity of this concept to the Platonic conception of love as generation in the Beautiful in the dialogue Symposion is clear. Life with a view of its comparative—"life transcending its own boundaries, is not something that comes to it from the outside. It is its own immediate being itself" (p. 295). So human striving for improvement and comparatives is not an accident but an essential basic condition of man.

The consumer industry seizes on the intentional human desire for improvement and implants it as meta-goods in advertisements of consumer goods and services: Viagra or skin creams make you younger, newspapers cleverer, dresses more beautiful, steel watches tougher, sports cars faster and deodorants olfactory and thus generally more socially acceptable. The advertising campaigns convey the order of comparative improvement to the potential consumer. They exclaim the *imperative of comparative melioration*: "Improve yourself!," "either better than you are so far or better than the others…" Such imperatives are above all found where advertising strategists believe that the consumer suspects a personal deficiency—in the areas of beauty, youth, health, spiritual, mental and physical energy or power, including sexual "performance."

3. Viagra and the Pathologization Disorder: A Diagnosis of its Symptoms

Pathologization prepares the ground for continuous comparative melioration. A healthy person is not necessarily in need of medical improvement, but nobody is really healthy nowadays. This is brought about by diverse negative side effects of today's lifestyles and its consumer culture on the one hand (malnutrition, lacking exercise, etc.) and by the strategy of pathologization on the other hand. Today's people are *a priori* in need of treatment. For the medical system and its paradigm of growth pandemics are essential for the survival of the system and this is exactly the reason why everyone is not healthy by definition, from birth to death.

The Western allopathic medical system seems to be signified by certain factors which make marketing of Viagra quite efficient. I am going to explain those factors more in detail in the following paragraphs. The factors include the pressure to generate wealth, non-holism and specialization, a mechanic understanding of the human biology and psyche, symptom treatment, "quick-fix"-treatments, deficiency in the concentration on health education and health consciousness, and a deficiency in initiatives for preventive care. These factors very much contribute to the marketability of popular antidepressants like Prozac or lifestyle drugs like Viagra.

Unlike in traditional tribal African or Asian medico-religious systems the Western health care system is also—and probably foremost—a wealth generating system with a fully fledged industry and its market and marketing campaigns in the background to which research programs and institutions are attached (and funded), which hardly contest this medical system. It is obvious that research sponsored by medical companies will not work in a direction which will make the whole system obsolete. Although some placebo research or the research findings about placebo control groups show that the "ritual" attached to the real medication is of high significance and sometimes as important as or even more important than the medication itself. In the case of Viagra 24% of patients, to whom placebos have been given also reported an improvement of their erectile function (cf. Pfizer website). Since the western concept of wealth is attached to the idea of growth it is also clear that the health care system has to continuously widen the notions of disease, sickness, and insanity or "disorder." While the jokes about the right and the left eye specialists and the "Monday morning getting up disorder" are still funny, the funny side of it disappears if one reads patients' entries into internet blogs about their "journeys" from one specialist to the next, each of them trying to classify a certain symptom within her or his area of specialization. Of course there are combinations of symptoms which give a clear-cut picture of a particular medical condition. But this is not always the case if one believes the experience of patients whose patience had been overstretched by wrong diagnoses and who at an advanced stage had become unintentionally self-made-specialists due to internet based exhaustive "research," being able to diagnose their own problem quite accurately and often some of them even "cured themselves." While this is not the standard in the Western medical system these "self-curing" attempts are definitely an interesting area of health research in line with Kant's notion of enlightenment according to which we should "have courage to use our own understanding" (1904, p. 35) instead of finding "a physician to determine my diet for me, and so on" (ibid.). In such a case "I need not think, if only I can pay: others will readily undertake the irksome work for me" (ibid.). While Kant, according to most of his biographers, was not overly successful in self-diagnoses and self-treatment (cf. Weischedel, 1993, pp. 170–180), this limited success could be attributed to the lack of sufficient information resources such as the internet, which in a way serves the spirit of enlightenment if used appropriately.

In the case of Viagra ED is conceptualized as *"a real medical condition"* which *"should be treated like one"* because *"in most cases, your erections won't improve without treatment"* (www.viagra.com/about-erectile-dysfunction/erectile-dysfunction.aspx). Nevertheless it is acknowledged that the reason for ED could be versatile (physical, psychological, social, circumstantial), the prescribed treatment is still the allopathic chemical "quick-fix." So Viagra usage is not a holistic, but an allopathic symptom-treatment leaving out any other alternative treatment. Viagra advertisements show openly (but communicate rather subliminally): 'if you feel as old as (or older than) you look like', 'if you partner is attracted to younger men', 'if you want to have fun beyond the forties', or *"if your thing is gone - but you want to ride on"* (Eric Clapton: Cocaine) there is only one possibility for revival: "Viva Viagra."

Related to the non-holistic approach of the mechanical Western system is its understanding of health in particular and biology in general. The prevalent view of humanity, especially in the bio-sciences, is a mechanical one, or at least one that is strongly influenced by physics. This has led to a one-sided concentration on the body, which is easier to explain via physical metaphors than the phenomenon of the mind, which in this monistic view of man is often regarded as a 'precipitate' of the body and that can ultimately be explained and treated according to physical rules.

From this follows that medico-therapeutic melioration of man mainly focuses on his physical nature and that his mental constitution is only treated as a second instance. Advertising strategists, being the more holistic 'therapists', have recognized this lack, which is why possibilities of mental improvement via meta-goods are included in advertising strategies. To speak cynically, it is possible to discern a 'therapeutic labor division' in Western societies: While classical Western allopathic medicine firstly deals with treating the body and places the psyche second, advertising has recognized the market lacuna 'melioration of the psyche' and filled it with meta-goods. In the case of ED Viagra does not only chemically lift what is physically down but this kind of body related melioration is also accompanied by mental, spiritual, and social elevation. This is also suggested by the adverts. While the reasons for ED in reality, and in the Viagra adverts, are versatile, the treatment is chemo-physical, but again the result is quite holistic and versatile: According to the adverts Viagra customers (and their partners) get younger, more attractive, happier, and more satisfied. It is quite interesting how the (potential) customers/patients are made to believe that a versatile problem can be transformed into holistic well-being and all-round satisfaction by a single blue diamond shaped pill, as if it were elderly men's best friend. But this quick-fixing symptom treatment via mechano-chemical means is symptomatic for the Western allopathic medical system so that the claim that this system is "unhealthy" in itself and making people sick (pathologic) might be a justifiable one. This is especially true if one considers that the system has significant deficiencies in terms of health education, health consciousness, and prevention for health. Although it is obvious that those characteristics are not entirely absent from the system it must be assumed that health prevention, consciousness, and education are from an economic point of view not very beneficial.

In sum it has to be stated that the Western medical system, aggregately seen, is suffering from a kind of maldevelopment or disorder—a pathologization disorder: To pathologize something which is not pathological for economical ends is in itself pathological. This is what I mean by pathological pathogenization. A related problem is that the side effects of this pathologization are pathogenic as well: Viagra and its adverts are pathogenic, in terms of (potential) physical side effects, if the pill is taken and in terms of psychological side effects if it is not taken; and maybe even if it is taken, because the man is not a full man anymore without Viagra. But logically seen the man is only a full man with it, according to Viagra adverts, and that does not remove the fact that in a "post-erectile age" the full man cannot exist anymore without medical assistance and somebody who essentially needs assistance is not capable of doing it on his own.

Having shown some of the characteristics of the Western medical system which make Viagra marketing successful I will now turn to demonstrate how this medical system attempts to continuously widen its scope of treatment.

4. Pathogenization as Viagra's Marketing Strategy

The strategy of extending the variety of products and services can increase the profit of businesses. This can either happen by offering more specialized products within a given product range, as it has been the case for example with sports equipment, or by widening the range of products, which happens if a company decides to offer products and services beyond their so far existing scope, as for example in the case of electronic products. The health care business is no exception. When comparing the processes of giving birth and dying in Western-style cultures on the one hand and developing countries' traditional (e.g. African) cultures on the other hand, we can easily see that usually birth/death take place at different places and are monitored and supported by different people depending on the respective culture. In modern Western-style societies birth and death usually take place in the environment of professional health care personnel, often in a hospital. In contrast, in rural areas in African cultures (as for example in the high mountains in Lesotho) birth and death are accompanied by a few cultural rituals in a private hut, surrounded by family members (in many cases without professional medical support). While the Western medical system clearly has advantages, in comparison to traditional medical systems, if it comes to emergency health care, the system's standardized procedures can be dangerous when for the sake of precaution and safeguarding too many medical strategies—with accompanying side effects—are employed, so that one side effect triggers a problem which has not existed in this shape before the intensive medical applications. The long and short term side effects of antibiotics (e.g. antibiotic resistance) and antidepressants (e.g. suicidal thoughts or change of personality) are often employed examples for this claim. Due to the professionalization of health care in Western-style cultures birth, ageing, and dying, which were normal processes in the life of a human being in traditional cultures, are meanwhile in most cases defined as 'medical conditions' which should be given professional medical attention. While there is nothing wrong in general with professional medical attention there might be a problem with the standardized (and thus almost compulsory) application of e.g. episiotomy and the giving of hormones for the initiation of birth, just to mention one example which can be observed in different cultures in which Western-style medical practices are prevalent.

The strategy of the medical system is not only to maintain its momentum of care, but also to intensify it and to extend its realm beyond simply curing diseases. An example of a fast growing branch within the rapidly expanding health care system is plastic surgery. It makes possible what is not achievable in the realm of cosmetics and beauticians: a permanent alteration of appearance (younger and/or more beautiful) following personal aesthetic ideals or fashionable trends. Also gender-reassignment must be seen in this context as well as the creation of the so called "third sex," the transgender person. In all those aesthetic and beauty health care issues comparative melioration plays a crucial role in marketing and decision making. But it should not be forgotten that now beauty and aesthetic ideals are no longer simply fashionable but medical issues. This is why we need beauty "therapists." There is a possibility to improve beauty with the help of the medical system. Beauty is therefore associated with health—and thus conditions which are potentially beautifiable are automatically associated with disease, sickness, and dysfunction.

Seen from this perspective the medical system is creating a new kind of sickness and dysfunction, it acts pathogenic. Potentially beautifiable persons are not as "healthy" as already beautified persons. The medical system indirectly equates beautifiable persons with unhealthy persons. Thus the system acts in a pathogenizing way, it creates new diseases: something like a "not-yet-beautified-disorder," which can be treated easily, by beautification. Another implication can be that someone who feels not beautiful enough might indeed get sick, at least psychologically. And in this way the medical beauty industry is in a position to create real psychological disorders which can be either treated professionally by psychologists or psychiatrists or can be better prevented by medical beauty surgery. But to make people sick for the sake of economic reasons is itself a severe disorder, therefore the system is also pathological (sick in itself).

The strategy of marketing Viagra is not that much different. ED is defined as a disease: if you don't do something against it you probably get also psychologically sick (pathogenic). And defining something which is "normal" as dysfunctional for the sake of making money is sick as well (pathological):

ED is also known as impotence. This equation bears several problems. ED is more specifically related to a particular bodily function while impotence is a wider term which can signify a general lack of power, force, and potentials but also sexual impotence. With this kind of rhetoric a specific physical "dysfunction" (an ED) is equated with a dysfunction encompassing the whole man. But what is even more striking is the following: if ED is related to age in such a way that statistically ED biologically or naturally increases with age, E "D" is a normal function of age and as such not a "dys"-function. And here we come back to the problem that age itself is turned into a dysfunction, which needs medical treatment.

5. Conclusion

This chapter's purpose was to enlighten the relation of the anthropological fact of comparative melioration and the pathological pathogenization of the Western medical system with the example of the ED medication Viagra and its marketing strategy. Pfizer is exploiting a philosophic-anthropological condition, that of comparative melioration, and at the same time pathologizing a natural function of age which is redefined as dysfunction. Viagra is another example of the combination of the comparative melioration and the pathogenization in Western health "care" marketing strategies. While the comparative melioration is an anthropological datum which we hardly can change and maybe do not want to change, even if we could, the pathologization is pathogenic and is not working for health care but against it. How lawmakers should act against the pathogenization strategy of the Western medical system is a question which cannot be followed further in this context. But the individual is in a position to emerge "from his self-imposed immaturity" (Kant, 1904, p. 35) and make the motto of enlightenment also a guideline in health care related issues: "Have courage to use your own understanding!" (ibid.). This is nowadays, if it comes for example to the issue of health care, easier than in the days of Kant, due to the availability of information via the internet.

An appeal to health care systems should be to place more emphasis on prevention, health education, and the promotion of healthy lifestyles in relation to exercise, nutrition, and social, psychological, as well as spiritual health.

Another philosophic-anthropological fact which has to be taken into consideration in the context of health care is the uniqueness of the human being in terms of biology, genetics, social-cultural, and psychological development, context, and circumstances. Certain medical normative suggestions which are appropriate for some must not be suitable for all. This of course also applies to sexual norms.

I close this paper with a suggestion, by combining the aforementioned Eric Clapton phrase from his song *Cocaine* with Kant's enlightenment demand:

"If your thing is gone" ... "use your own understanding!"[1]

Notes

1. Acknowledgments: The section on comparative melioration contains parts which are based on blended passages of chapter 2.2 from my book "Der Mode-Mythos" which has been translated by John Irons. All German quotations in those parts have also been translated by John Irons (johnirons.com). I wish to thank Taylor Hargrave for his critical comments and substantial suggestions which helped me to improve this paper.

Fifteen

ERECTUS INTERRUPTUS: ALL ERECTIONS ARE NOT EQUAL

Bassam Romaya

1. Preamble: The *Im*moral of the Story

Impotency drugs have been largely manufactured and marketed to a mainstream sexual audience obsessed with the diagnosis and treatment of what is currently known as erectile dysfunction. A predominantly heterosexual and aging clientele basis once accounted for the target audience which helped anchor Viagra's success soon after it became available to the public in 1998. Gradually, target audiences included a younger and more global clientele basis, propelled by a socio-cultural and medico-economic drive to improve or remedy the sex lives of mainstream populations impacted by impotence. Sexuopharmaceuticals have been largely developed with mainstream sexual function (or dysfunction) in mind, with any sideline effect among alternative or nonmainstream practices taking root as a result of its product, wholly unrecognized or unintended. The focus of this essay is not so much on the pervasive and often uncritically accepted ailment commonly described as erectile dysfunction; rather the aim is to assess Viagra's prospects for use by a particular type of transsexual population—female to male transsexuals, otherwise known as transmen. This essay examines the ways in which erectile roles and functions are interpreted and contextualized, in part through a systematic or multifaceted discursive process emphasizing productivity and reproduction, so as to fulfill specific social, cultural, economic, or nationalist roles and aims; ones in which the use of Viagra is legitimized and indispensable yet unsuitable for use by nonmainstream populations with medically-assisted genital reconstructions that undoubtedly challenge heteronormative demands and coital contexts, yielding a complex web of mores that maintain essentialist gender binaries and continually privilege male-born erections.

2. Inequality and Phallic Privilege: Challenges of Procreation and Productivity

It is easy to recognize that vast social, racial, ethnoreligious, and economic inequalities abound in contemporary industrialized societies (as well as non-industrialized ones of course). Without much fancy footwork, many have come to recognize that multiple inequalities resolutely persist in every sphere of modern social living. While much social justice and civil rights work has tirelessly worked to curtail common forms of rampant inequalities (viz., sexism, ageism, racism, and homophobia) throughout the past few decades, more subtle forms of social and sexual inequalities have persisted unchallenged. This is not due merely to persistent social injustices that remain unchecked or the continued presence of vulnerable or oppressed populations who have escaped efforts at securing reparations for past harms committed. In our times, subtler, multipronged, and marginalized inequalities reveal a social and sexual context in which non-dominant populations, particularly sexual subcultures, sexual minorities, transgendered people, and transsexual communities are continually disregarded in all facets of modern social living, or medically manipulated and pathologized once acknowledged.

As previously mentioned, Pfizer's initial target audience was the predominantly heterosexual aging male population eager to sample its product line. Gradually, the target audience became a younger generation of men, often with no recognizable erectile defects, men who use Viagra recreationally or as a result of the mistaken belief that the drug will strengthen or enhance their sexual experience; over the years, younger men (between 18-45 years of age) have come to account for the largest population base of the drug's users (Marshall, 2006, pp. 354-355). Apart from the visual presence of younger and younger men appearing in Viagra's advertisements, the drug gradually came to adopt a rejuvenating reputation, and ultimately, a recreational status along the lines of illicit party drugs (Vares and Braun, 2006, p. 328). The initial and subsequent target audience helped to secure the success of Pfizer's concoction. More importantly, the Viagra phenomenon, once defined by the sociologist Meika Loe as "a dynamic, tension-filled, ongoing and varied cultural movement, centered around a blockbuster drug and biotechnological product, which constructs and problematizes gender, sexuality, aging, and medicine" (Loe, 2001, p. 104), reinvigorated and reinforced vast inequalities that extend far beyond conventional critiques of phallocentricism, sexism, heterosexism, and ageism; championed by those working within the interdisciplinary domain of what gradually came to be known as "Viagra studies," incorporating an assortment of analytic tools derived from psychology, sociology, media studies, as well as gender, women and sexuality studies (Potts and Tiefer, 2006, p. 270). However, in all the Viagramania, and with minimal exceptions, no attention has been paid to the use (or prospects for use) across nonmainstream populations. Nonmainstream contexts in which Viagra plays a role have been predominantly focused on gay male populations (Vares and Braun, 2006, p. 328; Croissant, 2006, p. 336). Cisgendered males have, despite orientation or behavior, incorporated Viagra in various aspects of their sex lives.[1] While it is rather uncontroversial to recognize that the Viagra phenomenon has been part of gay male subcultures since its introduction to consumers, the drug has not similarly impacted other nonmainstream subcultures, such as lesbian communities for instance.[2]

The so-called Viagra phenomenon largely identifies sexual satisfaction with mainstream penile-vaginal heterosexual intercourse, namely coitus. What's more, heteronormative penetrative sex stands at the apex of norms and expectations, with climax (usually male climax) a pervasive and routine measure of virility or sexual effectiveness. On this model, the phallus is functioning in its idealized role as erectile, penetrative, and climactic—a phallic privilege bestowed upon the everyday heterosexual phallus derived from its potential role in fulfilling mainstream social expectations of productivity and procreation, with non-heteronormative variations on the theme seldom acknowledged or recognized. Phallic privilege is a byproduct of firmly entrenched value structures that intersect social, cultural, generational, religious, economic, and national mechanisms for prescribing cisgendered phallic roles and norms—ones which extend far beyond dutiful and socially-sanctioned sexual practice. Privileging the mainstream phallus fosters procreative endeavors among otherwise presumably frigid or unfruitful mainstream populations. It advances contemporary (and often neoconservative) American visions of procreative sanctity in the form of fruitful child-bearing and child-rearing families embodying divinely prescribed—though nationalistically and pseudo-theocratically ordained—multilevel social and sexual roles for the totality of its nationalist productive and procreative members. The roots of these multifaceted privileging structures are complex and far-reaching, for they extend across distant lands and ancient times. As early as the fifth century BCE, the Chinese philosopher Mo Tzu introduced the first recorded account of social, economic and political utility, long before Jeremy Bentham and John Stuart Mill formulized utilitarianism into a modern ethical theory. Mo Tzu's *nationalist* brand of utilitarianism vigorously espoused consequentialist objectives achieved through the means of population growth, social and economic productivity, as well as submission to state authority so as to ensure the greater good of the community. Unlike modern utilitarianism, the ancient Chinese thinker did not measure utility in psychological states such as happiness or pleasure nor in obtaining excessive luxuries for the greatest number, utility was measured in terms of economic productivity and prosperity, social and political stability, and fostering conditions that secure the basic needs of life (Cooper, 2003, pp. 74-80).

Apart from the interrelation between phallic privilege and mainstream procreative sensibilities, mainstream phallic norms are fashioned so as to increase personal and economic productivity. The strive to forestall or reverse the process of aging was once wholly concerned with reaping non-sexual rewards of youthfulness and rejuvenation—that is, the focus was once on regaining male vigor and productivity rather than male virility as it has recently become (Marshall, 2006, p. 347). Medical and public interest in male rejuvenation therapy throughout the early twentieth century was a byproduct of general trends that traced their roots to the American industrial revolution of the nineteenth century and increasing influence of capital markets in the early part of the twentieth century. Clinical interest in youthfulness and longevity was in part, motivated by a desire to increase work productivity. The decades of the great depression and the two world wars paved the way for commercial interest in extending and maintaining labor productivity, which once served as the principle factor motivating interest in age-defying or age-reversing biotechnologies. The circumstances surrounding current and widely-accepted privileging norms for cisgendered erections are bound up with long-standing and multifaceted nationalist, social, cultural, and economic utilitarian structures that value increased and improved bodily performance as well as the ability to procreate; two very crucial components that work together to privilege the heteronormative cisgendered phallus, seemingly lacking in nonmainstream phallic embodiments—namely, transerections.

3. Transmen, Transphobia, and Transerections

Theoretical complications abound in conceptualizing nonmainstream yet very real possibilities within both innate and reconstructed human anatomical diversity. Thus far, conventional analyses within the vast interdisciplinary domain now encompassing Viagra studies have produced a vast body of literature solely focused on the drug's use by biological males with cisgendered erections. As the search was on to pathologize female sexual "dysfunction" and ultimately to capitalize on a possible market for the pink Viagra, a host of theorists responded with critical accounts that examine the ways in which the pink pill—if at some point, it is fully developed, approved and marketed—stands to adversely impact the lives of cisgendered women. Impediments to developing the pink pill have been numerous, though not specifically due to any presumed differences between male and female physiology or sexuality; rather complications are a byproduct of misunderstanding both the nature and scope of sexual arousal, desire, and satisfaction: yielding the unenlightening conclusion that female (though ultimately male as well) sexual response is cognitively bound up with broader cultural dimensions and social contexts. That is, it is contextualized rather than robotic, having little to do with mechanistic genital function (Tiefer, 2003, pp. 3-4). The idea that context facilitates or contributes to arousal has broader implications; it underscores the importance of various external factors that may both hinder and enhance subjective sexual experience. Similar conclusions have been reached in other types of contextual experience; in recognizing the role of contexts while apprehending the natural environment or encountering an artwork. In the philosophy of art, influential contextualist theories maintain that social, cultural, historic, or biographical information is necessary to understand and thereby gain an appreciation for artworks, artifacts, or aesthetic objects.[3]Accordingly, human sexuality is often contextualized as well, combining introspective experience with real-world encounters that largely determine the success rate for an instance of sexual arousal. Though more to the point, female sexuality/ies are further complicated by considering the case of female to male transsexuals, in whole or in part, for whom cultural and social contexts come to play an even greater role in forming and shaping a chosen gender identity or sexual role, especially since transmen enjoy a sort of pansexualism, being "primarily attracted to males, other transmen, or masculine females" (Hansbury, 2005, p. 253). Absent from the slew of Viagra accounts is a consideration of the possibilities within an increasingly more visible and expanding universe of sexual and gender diversity—our paradigm case: transmen.

Female to male (FTM) transsexuals, often described as transmen, are usually lumped in with other nonmainstream populations with respect to sexual orientation or gender dysphoria. The vast body of work which has come to be described as GLBT (Gay Lesbian Bisexual Transgender) studies has only recently recognized the presence and contributions of female to male transsexuals.[4] Within this expansive domain encompassing GLBT studies, the focus has traditionally been directed at male to female (MTF) transgender-identified or postoperative transsexual women—transwomen for short. However, throughout the past two decades, FTM communities began to mobilize and take shape, building strong alliances both within and independently of the broader GLBT community. While transmen once solely relied on the Internet to network or obtain information unavailable in their communities, there are now more resources available, including varied support groups and other community-based outreach initiatives (Cline, 2004). Despite increased mobility and presence, the transmale population remains largely understudied. Academic attention has only recently awakened to the presence and emergence of transmen as a unique and worthwhile area of study—with most theoretical work still carried out by self-identified transmen themselves.[5] The overdue neglect of this population as an important yet distinct area of study was due in part to (real or imagined) attempts at prioritizing issues central to cisgendered men over concerns impacting the lives of cisgendered women; mimicking and perpetuating a male-dominated hierarchy that exists in every stratum of society—including GLBT communities. It is also important to note that issues of direct concern to transsexual communities are not identical to issues or causes championed by broader GLBT movements, this is but one of many reasons for distinguishing between the two populations; after all, transwomen are not hyperfeminine gay men and transmen are not stone butch lesbians.[6] Though GLBT and transcommunities often collaborate or politically mobilize in unison for the sake of resisting social oppression or seeking social justice, the unique and complex challenges that transmen encounter throughout their lives make transphobia a wholly different social disease than homophobia or say biphobia (Halberstam, 1998, p. 288). Additionally, while many transwomen and transmen initially seek support in the broader GLBT community, most eventually recognize the dissimilarities and differences between these groups, and ultimately seek out their own transcommunities. Of course, this is not to suggest that there is some unified transmale community to speak of here, since it is quite clear that intersectionalities cut across this loosely structured population group, just as multiple variations are present in other types of groups—it is expected that members differ by characteristics such as race, religion, class, or age. At one point it was common for transmen to make all the relevant changes so as to fully transition into men and blend into mainstream society. This usually includes going on testosterone therapy, having the relevant surgeries, changing one's name, and assuming a new identity. But times have remarkably changed. Many transmen are no longer concerned with reaping the rewards of passing privilege, by blending into the so-called "woodwork" (passing transmen are often called "woodworkers" for this reason) and becoming indistinguishable from cisgendered men. Blending into the woodwork and staying there, does not allow transmen to build solidarity with other transmen (or transwomen); further still, it does not aid in raising mass consciousness about the plight of transmen, nor does it allow for embracing and celebrating one's full transidentity (Hansbury, 2005, pp. 246-251). For this sense of internalized transphobia among transmen is out of date today.[7]

The lives of transmen offer a unique vantage point with which to conceptualize more subtle philosophical problems within the Viagra phenomenon. Transmen present a fundamental challenge to preconceived notions about gendered bodies and sexual identities; enabling them to play a crucial role in undermining essentialist and biological foundations that circumscribe all aspects of social, cultural, and nationalist norms (Cromwell, 1999, p. 43). The Viagra phenomenon has been frequently critiqued in the context of conventional usage by cisgendered heterosexual couples, forming the quintessential population base from which to analyze the phenomenon and jut forth studies examining its broader impact. Critiques of the growing phenomenon grew out of research informed by sociological, cultural, and medical backgrounds, as well as feminist-inspired critiques mainly from the United States and New Zealand, the only two countries thus far permitting DTC (direct to consumer) marketing of pharmaceutical drugs (Vares and Braun, 2006, p. 318). Accordingly, cisgendered male erections formed the data for all theoretical accounts mustered up in an effort to analyze and better understand the social dynamics, subtleties, and full range of complexities behind the phenomenon. While cisgendered male erections have been examined irrespective of the specific sexual roles they play (heterosexual, homosexual, or bisexual), no attention has been paid to the potential impact or effect of Viagra on non-cisgendered erections—namely, transerections.

Most readers are likely to be familiar with MTF transsexualism and perhaps some of the procedures involved in male to female gender reassignment surgery. Indeed this population is what many think of in conceptualizing or theorizing transsexualism. In postoperative male to female transsexuals, a series of surgeries from breast augmentation to vaginoplasty, culminate in the formation of a visually-convincing vagina suitable for penetration. Throughout the past century, male to female gender reassignment surgeries were more common to perform than female to male surgeries. Of course, this is not to suggest that transmen did not exist during that time (the high profile case of Billy Tipton comes to mind),[8] rather the lower incidence of female to male transsexualism was in part due to a lack of clinical awareness and medical technology available specifically designed for transmen, which only developed around the middle of the twentieth century—medically speaking, it has been easier to take off than add on, male genitilia. In the final decades of the twentieth century, further developments in female to male gender reassignment genital surgeries offered patients the means with which to fully transition into the gendered body they wished to inhabit. Apart from testosterone hormonal therapy, a variety of procedures are now available to aid patients in transitioning from female to male bodies, including bilateral mastectomy and chest reconstruction, as well as two main gender reassignment genital surgeries currently available for those wishing to make the full transition: 1) Phalloplasty and 2) Metoidioplasty. The first of the two options involves the surgical construction of a phallus using tissue taken from the forearm, side of the chest, abdomen, or groin area. The tissue is shaped into a tube resembling a phallus and grafted onto the patient's groin. The procedure commonly involves urethral extension (to enable standing urination) and tattooing the glans to simulate a phallus. Patients may also undergo other reconstructive surgeries such as vaginectomy, oophorectomy, and scrotoplasty, a procedure which involves the construction of male scrotum by extending and forming the tissues of the labia majora (a gradual process which may take several months to complete) and the insertion of silicone prosthetic implants proportioned in accordance with the patient's body. With phalloplasty, erections are only possible with the aid of an erectile prosthesis (a device similar to one used to treat impotence in cisgendered men) implanted only after the patient fully heals from phalloplasty. The second procedure, known as metoidioplasty, involves extending and repositioning the clitoris (enlarged as a result of long-term testosterone hormonal therapy) to form a very small phallus, or micropenis. Metoidioplasty may only be performed after the preoperative patient has been on testosterone therapy for a number of years, and the clitoris has expanded and lengthened considerably to allow for its surgical manipulation. Like phalloplasty, metoidioplasty is usually accompanied by scrotoplasty, as well as other reconstructive surgeries as needed. Since having the ability to void while standing is important for many transmen, both procedures allow patients to urinate while standing. Metoidioplasty may involve urethral extension (known as "metoidioplasty with urethroplasty") to enable urination while standing; though metoidioplasty may also be done without urethral extension. While both procedures are accompanied by their own set of advantages and disadvantages, metoidioplasty is usually the more attractive choice for many transmen purely for economic or practical reasons. Healing time is much shorter, the cost is substantially lower, and complications are fewer.[9]

While neither procedure offers patients a fully functioning penetrative phallus with naturally occurring erections, there are substantial differences between the two competing members. While phalloplasty results in a larger and more realistic looking penis, the neophallus itself is unable to achieve erections naturally, that is, without the assistance of a prosthetic device, at which point the neophallus becomes suitable for penetration. By contrast, the micropenis constructed as a result of metoidioplasty is able to achieve erections naturally without the aid of an internal prosthesis (which in any case, is not possible with metoidioplasty). Depending on the particular techniques used in releasing the clitoris from the pubis and repositioning it forward, genital sensation is often maintained and orgasm is possible with the resulting micropenis. Though the micropenis is able to achieve erectile functions naturally, it is far too small and tender to be suitable for penetration. While orgasm is possible with a micropenis, ejaculation is not, just as it is not possible for patients who have undergone phalloplasty.

Alas we have two distinct types of transerections to consider. While the neophallus is suitable for penetration, it is regrettably, unable to achieve erections naturally. Though the micropenis is able to gain erection naturally and independently, it is incapable of penetration. Neither of the two transerections is able to ejaculate—hence both are unable to inseminate or procreate. The very unique contemporary realities introduced by the neophallus and micropenis invite us to rethink essentialist and myopic social, cultural, or medical narratives perpetually inattentive to the range of sexualities and self-inscribed gender reconstructions, and equally oblivious to an expanding domain of erectile diversity.

4. All Erections Are Not Equal: Transerections Confront Viagra

While no conclusive data presently exists on the frequency of use or experimentation with Viagra by transmen, the subpopulation, with its resultant transerections, invites an extrapolation on or reconsideration of, formally held tenets with respect to Viagra's role in contemporary society. Moreover, it is important to entertain the possibility and attempt to connect missing links between Viagra's unparalleled success and its manufacturer's disinterest in reaching out to a marginalized yet potentially lucrative target market. At first sight, it may seem that the very limited market offered by the transpopulation in question is not significant enough to attract Pfizer's entrepreneurial attention. That is, dearth in consumer demand might initially account for the lack of corporate interest in providing a sexuopharmaceutical supply to meet the specific needs of transmen. Considering the broad margin for postoperative complications with female to male genital reconstruction surgeries, it stands to reason that a minute market may already exist, particularly for postoperative metoidioplasy patients, who are more likely to constitute the demand portion of the market equation. While the micropenis stands to benefit most from any enhanced sexual possibilities aided in the use of Viagra—notwithstanding its potential for enhancement—a micropenis is nonetheless unable to fulfill coital sexual norms cherished by Viagra and mainstream populations. To date, Pfizer has not invested research and marketing attention to alternative notions of erectile embodiment, function or dysfunction, nor is it likely to take into account these types of alternative configurations in prospects for future development.

Apart from attempting to carve out a potentially lucrative profit margin as a result of extending the reach of its economic tentacles deep into sexual subcultures, transgendered populations, and transsexual communities, the clinical and economic focus of Viagra has, all too predictably, been exclusively directed at the mainstream sociocultural level, with any variations remaining strictly at the level of cisgendered erectile dysfunction (or enhancement) frequently reported by gay or bisexual men (and this is the only nonmainstream audience that has made what might be viewed as *effective* use of the drug). The limited focus and understanding of the drug's capacity, magnitude, and fuller social or cultural ramifications invite a series of arduous questions. If it is the case that sexual satisfaction is solely gauged by the presence and frequency of coitus as the only route toward healthy, sustainable, and productive sexual lives, with no other combinations of relationships or sexual lives entertained or presupposed by Viagra's manufacturers (Vares and Braun, 2006, p. 324), how do very similar or even duplicate coital roles embodied and reenacted in the lives of many transmen become excluded from hegemonic standards by which normative coital relations dictate sexual health, purpose, and overall satisfaction? Put another way, since coital acts are possible via alternative reconfigurations involving transerections facilitated by developments in contemporary or postmodern biotechnologies, on what grounds does Viagra's manufacturer, Pfizer (and by extension other sexuopharmaceutical companies), come to exclude a target audience that *prima facie* replicates, appropriates, and reinforces heteronormative and often heteropatriarchal sociocultural or sexual roles that Viagra idealizes, extols, and exaggerates? How is it that Viagra comes to operate exclusively in a myopic context whereby coital acts facilitated by cisgendered erections serve as the only quintessential empirical model available for dictating corresponding paradigms that epitomize optimal sexual health? Part of the response has to do with erectile inequality.

The development and marketing of Viagra reveal in no uncertain terms a direct bias against non-cisgendered erections, setting up a false dichotomy in which transerections are deemed unworthy of equal sociocultural, sexual, and clinical consideration. In exposing, clarifying, and positing Viagra's discriminatory social and political stance, we do not mean to imply that erectile equality is a product of medically (that is *Viagrally*) enhanced erections; in other words, erectile equality is not empirically established by virtue of strength, length, or girth. Erectile quality itself is irrelevant in corresponding coital acts. Performing the act is what matters here, not the quality of genitals involved. The coital act itself (Viagrally-speaking) is the marker of satisfaction and otherwise healthy normative sexual lives. However, when similar or identical cases, coital acts in this regard, are treated differently, slighted, or dismissed by virtue of the identities or character traits found among participants, we may in fact conclude in no uncertain terms that all erections are not equal, even as competing erections participate in otherwise normative, standardized, heteronormative coital sex. Erectile inequality is a product of a transphobic disposition, an ill-intentioned disregard for the sexual lives of those whose transidentity disrupts, undermines, threatens, and emasculates otherwise genuine 'real world' cisgendered erections. On the conventional Viagra model, transerections are subverted through a process of systemic delegitimization, an erectile *ad hominem* if you will, one which frames the basis for attacking or dismissing the individual behind an erection (as opposed to the individual behind an argument) rather than judging his transerection solely on its own merit.

Let us revisit a point entertained in an earlier section. Interest in rejuvenation therapy throughout the past century was once partly motivated by efforts at increasing productivity, enhancing male vigor, and advancing nationalist procreative ideologies. In applying these and similar objectives to contemporary interests in propelling economic activity, productivity, and population increase, determinately and conveniently secured by various governmentally-sanctioned social and economic incentives to help build families, raise children, and fulfill a variety of social, cultural, governmental, and nationalist demands; in hindsight, transerections are rendered ill-suited for meeting the greater collective aims of increased economic productivity and procreation—this is the crux of the matter. It may be argued that transmen fall short of meeting multifaceted external demands that, in tandem, function so as to increase economic activity through the means of increased productivity. As a byproduct of their very limited numbers (rather than any particular shortcomings or traits shared among transmen), multifaceted external demands cannot be met through a sustained reliance on transproductivity, to actualize objectives aimed at increasing labor productivity.[10] It is not a simple matter to dismiss the usability, purpose, or functionality of transmen, and by extension, transerections, based on a line of reasoning which assumes that transmen fail to meet (dubious) external standards for meeting social and economic productivity. Recall that testosterone hormonal therapy is sometimes conceived as a *masculinizing* component associated with increased energy, improved work success, improved sexual desire, sports performance, and so on; that is, it may be argued that testosterone charged transmen may easily fulfill external demands of productivity merely in their everyday activities, just as testosterone therapy has been shown to help aging cisgendered men with improved vitality, greater professional competitiveness, increased energy and libido, so as to be more productive members of society well into their advancing years (Marshall, 2006, pp. 352-354).[11] Pervasive conceptions that promote ill-conceived notions of erectile inequality vis-à-vis lesser or decreased individual productivity are undoubtedly baseless, for they do not show a correspondence between transerections and lower productivity. Similar points contributing to erectile inequality might be advanced by emphasizing the general lack of transprocreation, or the perceived inability of transmen to reproduce, and thereby contribute to regional or global population growth. Of course, global overpopulation is a problem in itself, and no minimal lack of regional or national contribution is likely to hinder species propagation; the reverse, curbing population growth by avoiding unnecessary reproduction, is a more astute route toward greater utility.

It helps to note that developments in medical technology including reproduction and surgical techniques for transmen, are not always viewed favorably. Some have suggested that advances in science and technologies throughout the final decades of the twentieth century served to produce "cyborgian bodies" by creating a need for or dependence upon cutting-edge biomedicalization techniques that shape and structure, both gender and sexuality, as well as contemporary reproduction. For instance, Meika Loe notes that "postmodern techno-science scholarship suggests that transsexual, reconstructive, and cosmetic surgeries as well as reproductive technologies provide a window onto both social constructions and medico-technological interventions into gendered and sexualized personhood (…) where bodies are a collection of various parts, and sexuality is fractured and dispersed in and around the body, the surgeon's knife and hormonal treatments become tools for sexual enabling, reinvention, and goal-attainment" (Loe, 2001, p. 102). The gripe seems to be that the convergence of medical science and technology enables the creation, transformation, and trivialization of postmodern cyborgian bodies, genders, sexualities, and reproductive practices. The highly profitable medical market for gender reassignment surgeries as well as reproduction technology, attests to the commodification and commercialization of medical science and technology throughout the final decades of the past century and well into the twenty-first century.

Advances in reproductive technology aided by the development of sexuopharmaceutical drugs such as Viagra have streamlined and commercialized the coital procreative act such that reproduction comes to outline and reinforce essential functions of cisgendered erections. Viagra's capacity in aiding the act of conception was anticipated long before the drug became a reality, its very invention having emphasized its versatile role in both facilitating reproduction and fostering sexual intimacy (Croissant, 2006, p. 339). While transerections serve no reproductive role (recall that prosthetic testes are implanted and no ejaculation is possible with either metoidioplasty or phalloplasty), reproduction is often conveyed as a primary function for coital erections, bestowing phallic privilege exclusively on cisgendered erections busied with coital acts, leaving little room for transerections or the inclusion of other reproductive possibilities suitable for transmen, ones that do not rely on the hydraulics of transerections. Such a reproductive possibility is not too difficult to imagine; it is accomplished by forgoing bottom surgery, going off testosterone therapy, and choosing one of many artificial insemination methods available. While birth-giving remains a controversial practice among transmen, it leaves open the possibility for fatherhood, provided that transerections play no part (Hansbury, 2005, p. 253).

5. Conclusion: *Subsisto* Erectus Interruptus

In light of the forgoing juxtaposition among erections, and with little recognizable impact on increased productivity and no chance for procreation via transerection, what after all, is a transerection good for? While it may offer no utilitarian role in the conventional sense which cisgendered erections are believed to play, transerections are nonetheless *sui generis* creations imbued with their own sense of utility, in fostering individual well-being, completeness, or sexual satisfaction for those who possess and seek them. They need not be confined to gendered or sexualized roles, collapsed into the same oppressively limiting norms for cisgendered erections, nor any particular social, cultural, economic, nationalist, productive, or reproductive expectations. Erections across the board ought not be pathologized and bound up with distinct, utilitarian, or functional demands—most of all, they must not reap the benefits of phallic privilege, an underlying cause of erectile inequality.

The ancient and transcultural obsession with human erections, their size, function, quality, or purpose, is firmly entrenched in recorded history. It has dominated notions of masculinity, strength, superiority, and phallic beauty from the Romans and Ottomans to the Sadhus (Bordo, 2002, pp. 22-23). Foreshadowing a transfuture, Marquis de Sade once conceived fables of a turbulent world where cyborgian subjects sporting engorged superclitorises sodomize boys and men against their will.[12] But transerections must not be feared. They are by now a permanent part of our world, much as other variations, realities, or inventions of the imagination, such as aphrodisiacs, have undoubtedly become. The Colombian chef, Juan Sebastian Gomez recently created a "love dessert" made with the active ingredient in Viagra, a gendered dessert made exclusively for cisgendered erections. Such a culinary venture no doubt reinforces a variety of inequalities well beyond erections, despite claims to the contrary (Fairbanks, 2009). While the drug's manufacturer insists that Viagra is not an aphrodisiac and does not enhance erections or sexual experience for those not afflicted with impotence, its status as an aphrodisiac and recreational party drug is difficult to eschew (Vares and Braun, 2006, p. 327). Indeed, we are living the fictional future once widely feared, though seldom embraced: inhabited by cyborgs, genderqueers, transpeople and cisgendered impotents. A spectacular world enriched by difference is nothing to fear.

Notes

1. Cisgender may be thought of as the opposite of transgender. It simply describes biologically male or female bodies whose gender is aligned with behavioral norms socially or culturally prescribed for their particular gender. Female-born

and male-born heterosexual couples who initially formed the main consumer base for Viagra are individuals in cisgendered heterosexual relationships.

2. There are perhaps at least two reasons for this: first, by virtue of its mechanistic futility in the context of lesbian sex, and second, as a result of unsuccessfulness in developing a corresponding female Viagra—a dubious marketing and medical campaign viewed with much suspicion and hostility by many women, including self-proclaimed lesbians.
3. Modern contextualist theories may be contrasted with neo-Kantian isolationist accounts. Broadly construed, isolationists maintain that contexts corrupt the purity of aesthetic experience. In other words, artworks or aesthetic objects and events must be apprehended or understood apart from their particular histories, biographies, or particular contexts. For our purposes, Viagra implicitly operates on an isolationist basis, with little regard for the impact of sexual contexts. Contextualism may also be interpreted as a broader metaphysical view that combines elements of both idealism and realism. In other words, understanding the world in general involves reasoning through a historicized process that takes into account the past and present, as well as connecting the mind to the world, forming an anti-solipsistic disposition between our lives and their dynamic circumstances or surroundings. For an account of contextualism as an overall metaphysics, see the work of the Spanish philosopher Jose Ortega y Gasset in bibliography.
4. Sometimes the acronym is also known as LGBTIQ, which stands for Lesbian Gay Bisexual Transgender Intersex Questioning, with other combinations thereof likewise possible, depending on the author or categories to be grouped together. An elastic string of labels adds needless confusion and trivializes the topic under investigation. For instance, "Questioning" is not usually thought of as an identity nor do individuals in this group become the focus of an area of study within mainstream GLBT issues. And needless for mention, questioners (it is not at all clear what the questioner is questioning in the first place, apart from an expressed interest in sexual experimentation) do not share much in common with say, intersexed folks. Of course, Queer Theory is sometimes substituted as a convenient all inclusive umbrella term, but this is a misleading move since there are considerable differences within these fields of study that get lost when lumped together.
5. See for example the works by Jason Cromwell, Holly Devor (now Aaron Devor), Jamison Green, and Griffin Hansbury. Each author is a self-proclaimed transman (consult bibliography for full listings).
6. It helps to note that the "T" in GLBT studies refers to transgender, not transsexual. There is a great deal of dispute as to whether or not transsexual causes and issues should be included within GLBT concerns, particularly since issues of direct concern to transsexual communities bare little or no resemblance to issues of concern for the broader GLBT communities.
7. Raised on gender deconstruction, contemporary transmen are more empowered than ever before to feel free to inhabit the body they are most comfortable with. Some may choose to have "top surgery" but not "bottom surgery," take low doses of testosterone or forgo hormone therapy altogether, making them "lo-hos" or "no-hos." They may even choose to identify as "genderqueer" (an umbrella term encompassing the combinations or possibilities between gendered binaries) rather than transman.

8. Billy Tipton was an American jazz musician who reportedly married a woman and lived his life as a man, nearly 50 years of it. It was not discovered that he had female genitalia until his death in 1989. There is much dispute as to whether Tipton was in fact a lesbian forced to hide her sexuality in order to advance in a male dominated profession, or whether Tipton was in fact a transman falsely categorized as a lesbian (Halberstam, 1998, p. 293).
9. The price tag alone might make metoidioplasy the only option for many transmen, quotes range from $4,000 USD to $30,000 USD compared to a range between $100,000 to $150,000 for phalloplasty, a procedure which may involve multiple surgeries and increased recovery time (up to a year or more). Metoidioplasty has a higher success rate and is not subject to complications that arise from urethral extension (provided that urethroplasty was not performed) and device malfunction or migration associated with erectile prosthetic implants used by phalloplasty patients. Additionally, metoidioplasty often leaves less visible scarring (since no graft is involved) and it does not compromise functionality of the forearm or expose other parts of the body to the risk of infection, scarring, or other post-operative complications, especially if the graft area does not heal properly. For more detailed information about the latest in female to male transmedicine, see FTM International's website at: http://www.ftmi.org/.
10. There are exceptions worth noting: some might argue that transmen are quite capable of passing as men, joining a corporate workforce and vastly contributing to the proposed notion of social or economic productivity. I concur with the bulk of these claims. In fact, Griffin Hansbury describes his own experiences in the corporate world as a passing transman (Hansbury, 2005, p. 252–253). It may also be argued that the high cost of gender reassignment surgeries and continued medical attention that transmen may need, in conjunction with a lifetime of hormonal therapy, provide a new and very lucrative market that increases productivity as well as economic activity. Lastly, it is also well known that testosterone therapy itself contributes to increased energy and libido, and aides in the development of muscle tissue. These intuitions are indisputable, though they do not tip the scale in favor of erectile equality; this is essentially the matter at issue.
11. Barbara Marshall points out that over half of all men discontinue their treatment for erectile dysfunction as a result of waning sexual desire, in part brought on by "andropause," the male version of menopause, and its correlation with declining testosterone levels that develop naturally in men over the course of many years, especially in those over 50 years of age.
12. This theme appears in several of Sade's works, such as *The 120 days of Sodom*. Identifying the gender of Sade's characters is not always easy, since anyone (victims and rapists alike) might be sodomized by a phallic-sized clitoris or another object.

WORKS CITED

Adams, Christopher P. and Van V. Brantner. (2010) "Spending on New Drug Development," *Health Economics*, 19:2, pp. 130–141.

Al-Shaiji, T. F. and G. B. Brock. (2009) "Phosphodiesterase Type 5 Inhibitors for the Management of Erectile Dysfunction: Preference and Adherence to Treatment," *Current Pharmaceutical Design*, 15:30, pp. 3486–3495.

Althof, Stanley E. (2002) "Quality of Life and Erectile Dysfunction," *Urology*, 59:6, pp. 803–810.

———, et al. (1999) "EDITS: Development of Questionnaires for Evaluating Satisfaction with Treatments for Erectile Dysfunction," *Urology*, 53:4, pp. 793–799.

Ansell-Pearson, Keith. (1999) *Germinal Life: The Difference and Repetition of Deleuze*. New York: Routledge.

Appiah, K. Anthony and Amy Gutmann. (1996) *Color Conscious: The Political Morality of Race*. Princeton University Press.

Applbaum, Kalman. (2006) "Pharmaceutical Marketing and the Invention of the Medical Consumer," *PLoS Medicine*, 3:4, p. e189.

Aristotle. (1985) *Nicomachean Ethics*. Terence Irwin (trans.). Indianapolis: Hackett Publishing Company.

Aron, Raymond. (2001) *The Opium of the Intellectuals* [1955]. Piscataway, NJ: Transaction Publishers.

Arvon, Henri. (1973) *Stirner*. Paris: Seghers.

Augustine. (1910) *Confessions*. Edward Bouverie Pusey (trans.). Ithaca, New York: Cornell University Press.

———. (1948) *Soliliquies*. In *Writings of Saint Augustine. Vol. 1*.Translated by Thomas F. Gilligan. Washington, D.C.: Catholic University Press of America.

———. (1993) *On Free Choice of the Will*. Thomas Williams (trans.). Indianapolis: Hackett.

———. (1994) *City of God*. In *Nicene and Post-Nicene Fathers, First Series, Vol. 2*. Translated by Marcus Dods. Grand Rapids, MI: Eerdmans.

———. (1994) *On Marriage and Concupiscence*. In *Nicene and Post-Nicene Fathers, First Series, Vol. 5*. Translated by Peter Holmes and Robert Ernest Wallis. Grand Rapids, MI: Eerdmans.

———. (1994) *On the Good of Marriage*. In *Nicene and Post-Nicene Fathers, First Series, Vol. 4*. Translated by C. L. Cornish. Grand Rapids, MI: Eerdmans.

———. (1997) *Contra Julianum*. In *St. Augustine on Marriage and Sexuality*. Translated by Elizabeth Clark. Washington, D.C.: Catholic University Press of America.

———. (1997) Epistle 6 and 262. In *St. Augustine on Marriage and Sexuality*. Translated by Elizabeth Clark. Washington, D.C.: Catholic University Press of America.

Aversa, Antonio, Fernando Mazzilli, Tiziana Rossi, Michele Delfino, Andrea M. Isidori, and Andrea Fabbri. (2000) "Effects of Sildenafil (Viagra) Administration on Seminal Parameters and Post-Ejaculatory Refractory Time in Normal Males," *Human Reproduction*, 15:1, pp. 131–134.

Badinter, Elisabeth. (1986) *L'Un est l'autre*. Paris: Odile Jacob.

Bateson, Gregory. (1972) *Steps to an Ecology of Mind: Collected essays in Anthropology, Psychiatry, Evolution, and Epistemology*. San Francisco: Chandler.

———. (1979) *Mind and Nature: A Necessary Unity*. New York: Dutton.

Baudelaire, Charles. (1988) *Das Schöne, die Mode und das Glück – Constantin Guys, der Maler des modernen Lebens*. Berlin: Alexander Verlag.

Becker, Lawrence C. (1998) *A New Stoicism*. Princeton: Princeton University Press.

Benjamin, Walter. (1999) *Illuminations*. London: Pimlico.

Billerbeck, Margarethe. (1996) "The Ideal Cynic from Epictetus to Julian." In R. Bracht Branham and Marie-Odile Goulet-Cazé, ed. *The Cynics: The Cynic Movement in Antiquity and Its Legacy*. Berkeley: University of California Press.

Blight, David. (1985) "The Uncompleted Argument: Du Bois and the Illusion of Race," *Critical Inquiry*, 12:1, pp. 21–37.

———, and Robert Gooding Williams. (1997) "Introduction" to Du Bois.

Bloom, Allan. (1968) *Plato's Republic*. New York: Basic Books.

———. (1987) *The Closing of the American Mind.* Chicago: University of Chicago Press.

Boisaubin, Eugene V. and Laurence B. McCullough. (2004) "Prescribing Viagra in an Ethically Responsible Fashion," *Journal of Medicine and Philosophy*, 29:6, pp. 739–749.

Bordo, Susan. (2002) "Does Size Matter?" In Tuana, ed. pp. 19–37.

Botz-Bornstein, Thorsten. (2006) "Genes and Pixels: Popular Bio-Genetics' Virtual Aesthetics," *Angelaki*, 11:2, pp. 169–177.

Brisson, Luc. (2000) "L'incantation de Zalmoxis dans le *Charmide*." In Thomas M. Robinson & Luc Brisson, eds. *Plato Euthydemus, Lysis, Charmide. Proceedings of the Fifth Symposium Platonicum*. Sankt Augustin: Academia Verlag.

Brooten, Bernadette. (2003) "Nature Law and Custom in St. Augustine's on the Good of Marriage." In Shelly Mathews, Cynthia Briggs Kittredge, and Melaniwe Johnson-Debaufre, eds. *Walk in the Ways of Wisdom.* New York: Trinity Press International.

Brown Peter. (1988) *The Body and Society: Men Women and Sexual Renunciation in Early Christianity*. New York: Columbia University Press.

Burke, Cormac. (1990) "St. Augustine and Conjugal Sexuality," *Communio*, 17, pp. 545–565.

Butler, Judith. (2010) *Trouble dans le genre, trouble dans les normes*. Paris: La Découverte.

Caplan, Arthur L. (1989) "The Concepts of Health and Disease." In M. R. Veatch, ed. *Medical Ethics*. Boston: Jones & Bartlett, pp. 49–63.

Caponi, Gena Dagel, ed. (1999) *Signifyin(g), Sanctifyin(g), and Slam Dunking: A Reader in African American Expressive Culture*. Cambridge, MA: University of Massachusetts Press.

Carrick, Paul. (2001) *Medical Ethics in the Ancient World.* Washington: Georgetown University Press.

Castro-Vázquez, Genaro. (2006) "The Politics of Viagra: Gender, Dysfunction and Reproduction in Japan," *Body & Society*, 12: 2, pp. 109–129.

Chevret-Méasson, Marie, Emmanuel Lavallée, Sylvie Troy, Benoit Arnould, Séverine Oudin, and Beatrice Cuzin. (2009) "Improvement in Quality of Sexual Life in Female Partners of Men with Erectile Dysfunction Treated with Sildenafil Citrate: Findings of the Index of Sexual Life (ISL) in a Couple Study," *Journal of Sex and Medicine*, 6, pp. 761–769.

Chirac, Pierre and Els Torreele. (2006) "Global Framework on Essential Health R&D," *Lancet*, 367, pp. 1560–1561.

Cicero. (1923) *On Old Age, On Friendship & On Divination*. Cambridge: Loeb Classical Library.

———. (1956) *Letters to Atticus*. vol.1, E.O. Winstedt (trans.). Cambridge, MA: Harvard University Press.

Clark, Elizabeth. (1986) "Adam's Only Companion: Augustine and the Early Christian Debate on Marriage," *Recherches Augustiniennes*, 21, pp.139–162.

———. (1997) *St. Augustine on Marriage and Sexuality*. Washington, D.C.: Catholic University Press of America.

Cline, Elizabeth. (2004) "Transmale Nation: Remaking Manhood in the Genderqueer Generation," *Village Voice* (June 15).

Condry, Ian. (2006) *Hip-Hop Japan: Rap and the Paths of Cultural Globalization*. Durham: Duke University Press.

Conrad, Peter. (2007) *The Medicalization of Society: On the Transformation of Human Conditions into Treatable Disorders*. Baltimore, MD: Johns Hopkins University Press.

Cooper, David E. (2003) *World Philosophies: An Historical Introduction* Malden: Blackwell.

Crisp, Roger. (2009) "Well-Being." http//plato.stamford.edu/archives/spr2009/entries/well-being/ (accessed in February 2010).

Croissant, Jennifer L. (2006) "The New Sexual Technobody: Viagra in the Hyperreal World," *Sexualities*, 9:3, pp. 333–344.

Cromwell, Jason. (1999) *Transmen and FTMs: Identities, Bodies, Genders, and Sexualities*. Urbana: University of Illinois Press.

Daniel, G. Renigald. (1996) "Black and White Identity in the New Millennium: Unservering the Ties that Bind" in Maria P. Root, ed., *The Multiracial Experience: Racial Borders as the New Frontier*. Thousand Oaks: Sage.

Danoff, Dudley. S. (1993) *Superpotency: How to Get It, Use It and Maintain It for a Lifetime*. New York: Warner Books.

Darwin, Charles. (2005) [1859]. *The Indelible Stamp*. Philadelphia: Running Press.

Davis, F. James. (1995) "The Hawaiian Alternative to the One-Drop Rule" in Zack, ed.

De Grey, A.D.N.J., et al. (2002) "Time to Talk SENS: Critiquing the Immutability of Human Aging." In D. Harman, ed. *Increasing Healthy Life Span*, Vol. 959 of *Annals of the New York Academy of Sciences*. New York: The New York Academy of Sciences, pp. 452–462.

Dean, John et al. (2006) "Partner Satisfaction and Successful Treatment Outcomes for Men with Erectile Dysfunction (ED)," *European Urology Supplements*, 5, pp. 799–785.

———, Bert-Jan de Boer, Alessandra Graziottin, Dimitrios Hatzichristou, Jeremy Heaton, Ann Tailor. (2006) "Partner Satisfaction and Successful Treatment Outcomes for Men with Erectile Dysfunction (ED)," *European Urology Supplements* 5, pp. 779–785.

Del Casino Jr., Vincent J. (2007) "Flaccid Theory and the Geographies of Sexual Health in the Age of Viagra," *Health & Place*, 13, pp. 904–911.

DeLamater, John D. and Morgan Sill. (2005) "Sexual Desire in Later Life," *Journal of Sex Research*, 42 (May), pp. 138–149.

Deleuze, Gilles. (1988) *Bergsonism*. New York: Zone Books.
———. (1994) *Différence and Répétition*. New York: Columbia University Press.
Deng, F. M. (1972) *The Dinka of the Sudan*. New York: Richard and Winston.
Devor, Holly. (1997) *FTM: Female-to-Male Transsexuals in Society*. Bloomington: Indiana University Press.
Dinerstein, Joel. (1998) "Lester Young and the Birth of Cool." In Caponi, ed., pp. 239–278.
Diogenes Laertius. (1991) *Lives of Eminent Philosophers Vol. II*. Translated by R. D. Hicks. Cambridge: Harvard University Press.
Dorlin, Elsa. (2008) *Sexe, genre et sexualités: Introduction à la théorie féministe*. Paris: Presses universitaires de France.
Dortier, Jean-François, ed. (2008) *Les sex-toys, nouvel avatar de la luxure*, special issue of *Sciences Humaines*, 196, (August-September).
Du Bois, W.E.B. (1997) *The Souls of Black Folk*. Boston, New York: Bedford.
Dumas, Didier. (1990) *La sexualité masculine*. Paris: Albin Michel.
Durand, Gilbert. (1984) *Les structures anthropologiques de l'imaginaire*. Paris: Dunod.
Durham, W.H. (1991) *Coevolution, Genes, Culture and Human Diversity*. Stanford: Stanford University Press.
Edwards, D., et al. (2006) "Vardenafil Improves Sexual Function and Treatment Satisfaction in Couples Affected by Erectile Dysfunction (ED): A Randomized Double-Blind, Placebo-Controlled Trial in PDE5 Inhibitor-Naive Men with ED and their Partners," *Journal of Sexual Medicine*, 3, pp. 1028–1036.
Elliott, Carl. (2003) *Better than Well*. New York: Norton.
Elliott, Mark L. (1985) "The Use of 'Impotence' and 'Frigidity': Why has 'Impotence' Survived?" *Journal of Sex and Marital Therapy*, 11, pp. 51–56.
Engelhardt, H. Tristram, Jr. (1975) "The Concepts of Health and Disease." In H. Tristram Engelhardt, Jr. and Stuart F. Spicker, ed. *Evaluation and Explanation in the Biomedical Sciences*. Dordrecht: Reidel, pp. 97–121.
Epicurus. (1966) "Letter to Menoeceus." In Jason L. Saunders, ed., *Greek and Roman Philosophy after Aristotle*. New York: Free Press.
Fairbanks, Brian. (2009) "Viagra Desserts are Delicious and Trending Upward," *Asylum*, (November 16).
Farrer, James. (2010) "A Foreign Adventurer's Paradise? Interracial Sexuality and Alien Sexual Capital in Reform Era Shanghai," *Sexualities* 13:1, pp. 69–95.
Ferber, Abby L. (1995) "Exploring the Social Construction of Race: Sociology and the Study of Interracial Relationships" in Zack, ed.
Fishman, Jennifer R. (2004) "Manufacturing Desire: The Commodification of Female Sexual Dysfunction," *Social Studies of Science*, 34:2, pp. 187–218.
Fitzgerald, Mary. (2009) "Counting Cost of Cutting Aid," *Irish Times* (4 April). http://www.irishtimes.com/newspaper/weekend/2009/0404/1224243991197.html. Last accessed on 11 April 2009.
Foucault, Michel. (1976) *Histoire de la sexualité: La volonté de savoir*. Paris: Gallimard.
———. (1984) *Histoire de la sexualité II. L'usage des plaisirs*. Paris: Gallimard.
Frankenberg, Ruth. (1993) *White Women, Race Matters: The Social Construction of Whiteness*. Minneapolis: University of Minnesota Press.
Freud, Sigmund (2005) *Civilization and its Discontents*. New York: Norton.
———. (1905) *Le mot d'esprit dans ses rapports à l'inconscient*. Paris: Gallimard.

———. (1910) *Trois essais sur la théorie de la sexualité*. Paris: Payot.
———. (1912) *La peur de l'inceste dans Totem et tabou*. Paris: Payot.
———. (1915) *Métapsychologie*. Paris: Gallimard.
———. (1924) *Essais de psychanalyse III*. Paris: Payot.
Galen. (1976) *On the Affected Parts*. Translation from the Greek Text with Explanatory Notes by Rudolph E. Siegel, MD. Basel: S. Sarger AG.
Gehlen, Arnold. (1993) *Anthropologische und sozialpsychologische Untersuchungen*. Hamburg: Rowohlt.
Genet, Jean. (1948) *Notre-Dame-des-Fleurs*. Paris: Livre de poche.
Giles, Freda Scott. (1995) "From Melodrama to the Movies" in Zack, ed.
Gillis, Stacy. (2005) *The Matrix Trilogy: Cyberpunk Reloaded*. London, New York: Wallflower Press.
Global Forum for Health Research. (2004) *The 10/90 Report on Health Research 2003–2004*. Geneva: Global Forum for Health Research. http://www. globalforumhealth.org. Last accessed on 12 December 2010.
Glowka, Wayne, Katherine A. Bonner, and Brenda K. Lester. (1999) "Among the New Words," *American Speech*, 74:1, pp. 71–94.
Goldberg, David Theo. (1995) "Made in the USA: Racial Mixing 'n Matching" in Zack, ed.
Goldberg, Kenneth A. (1998) *Viagra: The Potency Pill*. Lincolnwood, IL: Publications International.
Goulet-Cazé, Marie-Odile. (1996) "Religion and the Early Cynics." In R. Bracht Branham and Marie-Odile Goulet-Cazé, ed. *The Cynics: The Cynic Movement in Antiquity and Its Legacy*. Berkeley: University of California Press.
Green, Jamison. (2005) "Part of the Package: Ideas of Masculinity among Male-Identified Transpeople," *Men and Masculinities*, 7:3 (January), pp. 291–299.
Haber, Carole. (1983) *Beyond Sixty-Five: The Dilemma of Old Age in America's Past*. New York: Cambridge University Press.
Halberstam, Judith. (1998) "Transgender Butch: Butch/FTM Border Wars and the Masculine Continuum," *GLQ: Journal of Lesbian and Gay Studies*, 4:2, pp. 287–310.
———. (1998) *Female Masculinity*. Durham: Duke University Press.
Handy, Bruce. (1998) "The Viagra Craze," *Time* (4 May), pp. 50–57.
Hansbury, Griffin. (2005) "The Middle Men: An Introduction to the Transmasculine Identities," *Studies in Gender and Sexuality*, 6:3, pp. 241–264.
Haraway, Donna J. (2008) *When Species Meet*. Minneapolis: University of Minnesota Press.
Hartley, Heather. (2006) "The 'Pinking' of Viagra Culture: Drug Industry Efforts to Create and Repackage Sex Drugs for Women," *Sexualities*, 9:3.
Hatzimouratidis, K. and D. G. Hatzichristou. (2009) "Phosphodiesterase Type 5 Inhibitors: Unmet Needs," *Current Pharmaceutical Design*, 15:30, pp. 3476–3485.
Hegel, W. F. (1939) *Phénoménologie de l'esprit*. Translated by J. Hyppolite. Paris: Aubier.
Held, René R. (1970) *Psychothérapie et psychanalyse*. Paris: Payot.
Helford, Elyce Rae, ed. (2000) "Introduction" to *Fantasy Girls: Gender in the New Universe of Science Fiction Television*. Lanham: Rowman & Littlefield.
Hershel, Helena Jia. (1995) "Therapeutic Perspectives on Biracial Formation" in Zack, ed.
Hesnard, Angelo. (1959). *La sexologie*. Paris: Payot.

Hillman, Jennifer. (2008) "Sexual Issues and Aging Within the Context of Work With Old Adult Patients," *Professional Psychology: Research and Practice*, 39:3, pp. 290–297.

Hippocrates. (1984) *Hippocratic Writings*. G.E.R. Lloyd, ed. & J. Chadwick (trans.) New York: Penguin Classics.

Hobbes, Thomas. (1998) *Leviathan*. New York: Oxford University Press.

Horney, Karen. (1967) *La psychologie de la femme*. Paris: Payot.

Hume, David. (1975) *Enquiries Concerning Human Understanding and Concerning the Principles of Morals, Third Edition* [1777]. Selby-Bigge, ed. Los Angles & Oxford: Oxford University Press.

———. (2005) *A Treatise of Human Nature* [1739,1740]. New York: Barnes and Noble.

Hunter, David. (1994) "Augustinian Pessimism? A New Look at Augustine's Teachings on Sex Marriage and Celibacy," *Augustinian Studies*, 25, pp.153–177.

———. (1999) "Marriage." In Allan Fitzgerald, ed. *Augustine Through the Ages*. Grand Rapids, MI: Eerdmans.

Hussein, Jeylan W. (2005) "The Social and Ethno-Cultural Construction of Masculinity and Femininity in African Proverbs" in *African Study Monograph*, 26:2 (August), pp. 59–87.

Irigaray, Luce. (1985) *This Sex which is not One*. Ithaca, New York: Cornell University Press.

Irvine, William. (2009) *A Guide to the Good Life: The Ancient Art of Stoic Joy*. New York: Oxford University Press.

Javet, Pierre. (1982) "Céphale et Platon sur le seuil de la vieillesse. Réflexions sur le prologue de la *République*," *Revue Philosophique*, 107, pp. 241–247.

Kaiser, Fran E. (1999) "Erectile Dysfunction in the Aging Man," *The Aging Male Patient*, 83:5 (September), pp. 1267–78.

Kakridis, Johannes Th. (1948) "The Part of Cephalus in Plato's *Republic*," *Eranos*, 46.

Kant, Immanuel. (1904) "Was ist Aufklärung" in *Kants gesammelte Schriften* (Akademie Ausgabe) Vol. 8. Berlin & Leipzig: De Gruyter.

———. (1983) *Perpetual Peace and Other Essays*. Indianapolis: Hackett Publishing.

Kass, Leon R. (1985) *Toward a More Natural Science*. New York: Free Press.

Katz, Stephen and Barbara Marshall. (2003) "New Sex for Old: Lifestyle, Consumerism and the Ethics of Aging Well," *Journal of Aging Studies*, 17, pp. 3–16.

———. (2004) "Is the Functional 'Normal'? Aging, Sexuality and the Bio-Marketing of Successful Living," *History of the Human Sciences*, 17:1 (2004), pp. 53–75.

Kerr, M. E. (1988) *Family Evaluation: An Approach Based on Bowen Theory*. New York: Norton.

Khayat, M. H. (no date) "Spirituality in the Definition of Health: The World Health Organization's Point of View." http://www.medizin-ethik.ch/publik/spirituality_definition_health.htm. Last accessed on 12 December 2010.

Kierkegaard, Søren. (1983) *Fear and Trembling: Repetition* [1843]. Princeton: Princeton University Press.

———. (2008) *Sickness unto Death* [1849]. Radford, VA: Wilder.

Kochman, Thomas, ed. (1972) *Rappin' and Stylin' Out. Communication in Urban Black America*. Chicago: University of Illinois Press.

———. (1981) *Black and White Styles in Conflict*. Chicago: University of Chicago Press.

Kojève, Alexandre. (1969) *Introduction to the Reading of Hegel* [1947]. New York: Basic Books [1947].
Konstantinos, Giannitsas and Perimenis Petros. (2009) "Phosphodiesterase-5 Inhibitors: Future Perspectives," *Current Pharmaceutical Design*, 15:30, pp. 3540–3551.
Kouvelas, D., A. Goulas, G. Papazisis, C. Sardeli, and C. Pourzitaki. (2009) "PDE5 Inhibitors: *In Vitro* and *In Vivo* Pharmacological Profile," *Current Pharmaceutical Design*, 15:30, pp. 3464–3475.
Kuhn, Thomas S. (1996) *The Structure of Scientific Revolutions, Third Edition*. Chicago: The University of Chicago Press.
Lacan, Jacques. (1971) *Ecrits I*. Paris: Seuil.
———. (1973) *Ecrits II*. Paris: Seuil.
———. (1984) *Séminaire XI: Les quatre concepts fondamentaux de la psychanalyse*. Paris: Seuil.
———. (2001) *Autres Ecrits VI*. Paris: Seuil.
———. (2005) *Séminaire XXIII: Le sinthome*. Paris: Seuil.
Lafontaine, Céline. (2009) "Regenerative Medicine's Immortal Body: From the Fight against Ageing to the Extension of Longevity," *Body & Society*, 15:4, pp. 53–66.
Laplanche, Jean and J. B. Pontalis. (1967) *Vocabulaire de la psychanalyse*. Paris: Presses universitaires de France.
———. (1976) "Phallus." In *Dictionnaire de la psychanalyse* (5th edition). Paris: Presses universitaires de France.
Leland, John. *Hip: The History*. (2005) New York. Harper Collins.
Lessenger, James E. and Steven D. Feinberg. (2008) "Abuse of Prescription and Over-the-Counter Medications," *Journal of the American Board of Family Medicine*, 21:1 (January-February), pp. 45–54.
Levine, Bruce E. (2001) "Commonsense Rebellion: Debunking Psychiatry, Confronting Society," New York: Continuum.
Lévi-Strauss, Claude. (1975) *Histoire de Lynx*. Paris: Plon.
Lexchin, Joel. (2006) "Bigger and Better: How Pfizer Redefined Erectile Dysfunction," *PLoS Med*, 3:4 (April), pp. 429–432.
Lidz, Joel W. (1995) "Medicine as Metaphor in Plato," *The Journal of Medicine and Philosophy*, 20, pp. 527–541.
Limin, Ma, Niels Johnsen, and Wayne J. G. Hellstrom. (2010) "Avanafil, A New Rapid-onset Phosphodiesterase 5 Inhibitor for the Treatment of Erectile Dysfunction," *Expert Opinion on Investigational Drugs*, 19:11, pp. 1427–1437.
Lipton, Peter. (1991) *Inference to the Best Explanation*. New York: Routledge.
Llewellyn-Jones, Derek. (1987) *Every Man*. Oxford: Oxford University Press.
Loe, Meika. (2001) "Fixing Broken Masculinity: Viagra as a Technology for the Production of Gender and Sexuality," *Sexuality and Culture*, 5:3, pp. 97–125.
———. (2004) "Sex and the Senior Woman: Pleasure and Danger in the Viagra Era," *Sexualities*, 7:3, pp. 303–326.
———. (2004) *The Rise of Viagra: How the Little Blue Pill Changed Sex in America*. New York University Press.
Long, A.A. (1996) "The Socratic Tradition: Diogenes, Crates, and Hellenistic Ethics." In R. Bracht Branham and Marie-Odile Goulet-Cazé, ed. *The Cynics: The Cynic Movement in Antiquity and Its Legacy*. Berkeley: University of California Press.

MacIntyre, Alasdair. (1984) *After Virtue: A Study in Moral Theology*. Notre Dame: University of Notre Dame Press.

MacKinnon, Grace D. (2004) "Is Using Viagra Immoral?"in *Catholic Exchange* September 28. Available at: http://catholicexchange.com/2004/09/28/82190.

Madigan, Timothy. (2008) "The Ancient Cynics: The First Environmentalists," *Philosophy Now: A Magazine of Ideas*, 68 (January-February).

Magesa, L. (1997) *African Religion: The Moral Traditions of Abundant Life*. New York: Orbis.

Mailer, Norman. (1970) *The White Negro: Superficial Reflections on the Hipster* [1957]. San Francisco: City Lights Books.

Majors, Richard and Janet Mancini Billson. (1992) *Cool Pose: The Dilemma of Black Manhood*. New York: Lexington Press.

Mamo, Laura and J. R. Fishman. (2001) "Potency in All the Right Places: Viagra as a Technology of the Gendered Body," *Body & Society*, 7:13, pp. 13–35.

Marcano, Donna-Dale. (2003) "Sartre and the Construction of Race" in R. Bernasconi, ed., *Race and Racism in Continental Philosophy*. Bloomington: Indiana University Press, pp. 214–226.

Marion, Jean-Luc. (2007) *The Erotic Phenomenon*. Chicago: University of Chicago Press.

Marshall, Barbara L. (2002) "'Hard Science': Gendered Constructions of Sexual Dysfunction in the 'Viagra Age'," *Sexualities*, 5:2, pp. 131–158.

———. (2006) "The New Virility: Viagra, Male Aging and Sexual Function," *Sexualities*, 9, pp. 345–362.

———, and Stephen Katz. (2002) "Forever Functional: Sexual Fitness and the Ageing Male Body," *Body & Society*, 8:4, pp. 43–70.

McGinn, Daniel. (1998) "Viagra's Hothouse," *Newsweek*, 132:25 (December 21), pp. 44–46.

McLaren, Angus. (2007) *Impotence: A History*. Chicago: University of Chicago Press.

Meilaender, Gilbert. (2001) "Sweet Necessities: Food, Sex, and Saint Augustine," *Journal of Religious Ethics*, 29:1, pp. 3–18.

Meinhold, Roman. (1997) "Meta-Goods in Fashion-Myths: Philosophico-Anthropological Implications of Fashion," *Prajna Vihara: Journal of Philosophy and Religion*, 8:2, pp. 1–15.

———. (2005) *Der Mode-Mythos: Lifestyle als Lebenskunst: Philo-sophisch-anthropologische Implikationen der Mode*. Würzburg: Königshausen & Neumann.

———. (2009) "Popular Culture and Consumerism: Mediocre, (Schein-) Heilig and Pseudo-Therapeutic." In: Yusuf, Imtiyaz and Canan Atilgan, ed., *Religion, Politics and Globalization. Implications for Thailand and Asia*. Bangkok: Konrad Adenauer Foundation.

Ménissier, Thierry. (1995) "Platon et la maladie dans la *République*," *Les Études philosophiques*, 50, pp. 355–373.

Merleau-Ponty, Maurice. (1962) *Phenomenology of Perception*. New York: Routledge.

Miles, Margaret. (2005) "Sex and the City (of God): Is Sex Forfeited of Fulfilled in Augustine's Resurrection of Body?" *Journal of the American Academy of Religion*, 73:2 (June), pp. 307–327.

Mill, John Stuart. (1998) *Utilitarianism* [1863]. R. Crisp, ed. Oxford: Oxford University Press.

Morales, K., T. Campos T, C.A. Roselli et al. (2005) "Erectile Dysfunction," *SMBJ*, 13, 441–484.

Morgentaler, Abraham. (1999) "Male Impotence," *Lancet*, 354, pp. 1713–18.

Moynihan, Ray and David Henry. (2006) "The Fight against Disease Mongering: Generating Knowledge for Action," *PLoS Medicine*, 3:4, p. e191.

Murphy, David J. (2000) "Doctors of Zalmoxis and Immortality in the *Charmides*." In Thomas M. Robinson & Luc Brisson, ed. *Plato Euthydemus, Lysis, Charmides. Proceedings of the V Symposium Platonicum*). Sankt Augustin: Academia Verlag.

Nails, Debra. (2002) *The People of Plato. A Prosopography of Plato and Other Socratics* Indianapolis: Hackett.

Nakamura, Lisa. (2005) "The Multiplication of Difference in Post-Millennial Cyberpunk Film: The Visual Culture of Race in the Matrix Trilogy," in Gillis, ed.

Navia, Luis E. (2005) *Diogenes the Cynic*. Amherst: Humanity Books.

Nicholls, E. Henry. (2003) "Andropause for Thought," *Endeavor*, 27:3, p. 99.

Nietzsche, Friedrich W. (1994) *On the Genealogy of Morality*. New York: Cambridge University Press.

NIH Consensus Development Panel on Impotence. (1993) "NIH Consensus Conference: Impotence," *Journal of the American Medical Association*, 270:1, pp. 83–90. Odeyemi, John Segun. (2004) *Catholics and Human Sexuality: The Humane Vitae Questions*. Iperu Remo: The Ambassador Publications.

Nozick, Robert. (1989) *The Examined Life*. New York: Simon and Schuster.

O'Mathúna, Dónal P. (2000) "The Goals of Medicine: The Case of Viagra." In John F. Kilner, Paige C. Cunningham, and W. David Hager, ed. *The Reproductive Revolution: A Christian Appraisal of Sexuality, Reproductive Technologies, and the Family*. Grand Rapids, MI: Eerdmans, pp. 46–59.

Okeregbe, Anthony. (2008). "The Nature of the Human Mind" in Godwin Azenabor ed. *Philosophical Psychology: Selected Readings*. Lagos: Promocomms Ltd.

Oloruntoba-Oju, Taiwo. (2009) "Body Image, Beauty, Culture and Language in the Nigerian African Context" in *Sexuality in Africa Magazine*, 5:4.

Omolade, Barbara. (1995) *The Rising Song of African American Women*. New York: Routledge.

Onfray, Michel. (2010) *Le crépuscule d'une idole*: *L'affabulation freudienne*. Paris: Grasset.

Otten, Willemien. (1998) "Augustine on Marriage Monasticism, and the Community of the Church," *Theological Studies*, 59, pp.385–405.

Pagels, Elaine. (1988) *Adam, Eve, and the Serpent*. New York: Random House.

Pang, Tikki, Ariel Pablos-Mendez, and Carel Usselmuiden. (2004) "From Bangkok to Mexico: Towards a Framework for Turning Knowledge into Action to Improve Health Systems," *Bulletin of the World Health Organization*, 82:10, pp. 720–722.

Parens, Erik. (1998) "Is Better Always Good? The Enhancement Project," *Hastings Center Report*, 28, pp. S1–S16.

Perelman, Michael A. (2001) "The Impact of the New Sexual Pharmaceuticals on Sex Therapy," *Current Psychiatry Reports*, 3:3, pp. 195–201.

Perkinson, Jim. (2002) "The Body of White Space: Beyond Stiff Voices, Flaccid Feelings and Silent Cells" in Tuana, ed.

Persons, Stow. (1975) *American Minds: A History of Ideas*. Huntington: Krieger.

Plante, Rebecca F. (2006) "Review of Meika Loe, *The Rise of Viagra: How the Little Blue Pill Changed Sex in America*," *Sexualities*, 9:3, pp. 137–140.
Plato. (1992) *Republic*. Translated by G.M.A. Grube. Indianapolis: Hackett.
———. (1997) *Complete Works*, ed. John M. Copper, Indianapolis: Hackett.
Pogge, Thomas W. (2005a) "Human Rights and Global Health: A Research Program," *Metaphilosophy*, 36:1/2, pp. 182–209.
———. (2005b) "Real World Justice," *Journal of Ethics*, 9, pp. 29–53.
———. (2008) *World Poverty and Human Rights*. Cambridge: Polity Press.
Potts, Annie and Leonore Tiefer. (2006) "Introduction" to *Sexualities* 9:3, pp. 267–272.
Potts, Annie, Nicola Gavey, Victoria Grace, and Tiina Vares. (2003) "The Downside of Viagra: Women's Experiences and Concerns," *Sociology of Health & Illness* 25:7, pp. 697–719.
———. (2004) "'Viagra Stories': Challenging 'Erectile Dysfunction'," *Social Science & Medicine*, 59, pp. 489–499.
Potts, Annie. (2004a) "Viagra Cyborgs: Creating 'Better Manhood' Through Chemistry?" In Potts et al., eds. *Sex and the Body*, Palmerston North, New Zealand: Dunmore Press.
———. (2004b) "Deleuze on Viagra (Or What Can a 'Viagra Body' Do?)," *Body and Society*, 10:1, pp. 17–36.
———. (2005) "Cyborg Masculinity in the Viagra Era." In *Sexualities, Evolution & Gender*, 7:1, pp. 3–16.
———. (2008) "The Female Sexual Dysfunction Debate: Different 'Problems', New Drugs—More Pressures?," *Contesting Illness: Processes and Practices*, Pamela Moss and Katherine Teghtsoonian, eds. Toronto: University of Toronto Press.
Pountain, Dick and David Robins. (2000) *Cool Rules: Anatomy of an Attitude*. London: Reaktion Books.
Power, Kim. (1996) *Veiled Desire: Augustine on Women*. New York: Continuum.
Price, Connie C. (2006) "Energy and Philosophy, An Appeal for Affective Justice," given at the 16th Annual Congress of *The International Association, Cosmos and Philosophy*," Novi Sad, Serbia.
Protevi, John. (2009) *Political Affect: Connecting the Social and the Somatic*. Minneapolis: University of Minnesota Press.
Quennell, Peter. (1988) *The Pursuit of Happiness*. Oxford: Oxford University Press.
Quinby, Lee. (1999) "Virile-Reality: From Armageddon to Viagra," *Signs*, 24:4, pp. 1079–1087.
Ramsay, Sarah. (2001) "No Closure in Sight for the 10/90 Health-research Gap," *Lancet*, 358, p. 1348.
Rauscher, Josef (2000) "Homo faber fabricatus. Aspekte eines neuen Menschenbildes aus dem Geiste des Designs," *Eine Zeit-Schrift für Alle. Interdisziplinäre Bildung und praktische Philosophie*, 3, pp. 10–18.
Reeve, C.D.C. (1988) *Philosopher-Kings. The Argument of Plato's* Republic. Princeton: Princeton University Press.
Rennie, Stuart and Bavon Mupenda. (2008) "Living Apart Together: Reflections on Bioethics, Global Inequality and Social Justice," *Philosophy, Ethics, and Humanities in Medicine* 3: p. 25.
Revel, Jean-Francois, and Matthieu Ricard. (1998) *The Monk and the Philosopher*. New York: Schocken Books.
Rist, John. (1996) *Stoic Philosophy*. Cambridge: Cambridge University Press.

Rosen, Raymond C., et al. (1997) "The International Index of Erectile Function (IIEF): A Multidimensional Scale for Assessment of Erectile Dysfunction," *Urology*, 49:6, pp. 822–828.

Rosen, Raymond C. (1998) "Sildenafil: Medical Advance or Media Event?" *Lancet*, 351, pp. 1599–1600.

Rosen, Stanley. (2005) *Plato's Republic. A Study*. New Haven: Yale University Press.

Rosolato, Guy. (1967) "Etude des perversions sexuelles à partir du fétichisme." In Valabrega et al., eds. *Le désir et la perversion*. Paris: Seuil.

Rubin, Henry. (2003) *Self-Made Men: Identity and Embodiment among Transsexual Men*. Nashville: Vanderbilt University Press.

Rubin, Naomi and Kevan Wylie. (2009) "Should Sildenafil be Available over the Counter?" *British Medical Bulletin*, 90, pp. 53–62.

Rubio-Aurioles, Eusebio, et al. (2006) "Comparing Vardenafil and Sildenafil in the Treatment of Men with Erectile Dysfunction and Risk Factors for Cardiovascular Disease: a randomized, Double-Blind, Pooled Crossover Study," *Journal of Sexual Medecine*, 3, pp. 1037–1049.

Ryan, Marie-Laure. (2001) *Narrative as Virtual Reality: Immersion and Interactivity in Literature and Electronic Media*. Baltimore: University of John Hopkins Press.

Ryff, Carol and Burton Singer. (2006) "Know Thyself and Become What You Are: A Eudaimonic Approach to Psychological Well-Being," *Journal of Happiness Studies*, 9:1, pp. 13–39.

Sabin, J. E. and N. Daniels. (1994) "Determining 'Medical Necessity' in Mental Health Practice," *Hastings Center Report*, 24:6, pp. 5–13.

Sacred Congregation for the Doctrine of the Faith, *Donum Vitae, Instruction on the Respect for Human Life in its Origin and on the Dignity of Procreation: Replies to Certain Questions of the Day*, 22 February 1987, *n.* II, A, 1: *AAS* 80 1988, 70–102.

Sade, Jean-Baptiste de. (1965) *The Complete Justice, Philosophy in the Bedroom, and Other Writing*. New York: Grove Press. French: *La Philosophie dans le boudoir*. Paris: C. Bourgois, 1998.

———. (1990) "Philosophy in the Bedroom." In *Justine, Philosophy in the Bedroom, and other writings*. Translated by Richard Seaver & Austryn Wainhouse. New York: Grove Press.

Safouan, Moustapha. (1976) *La sexualité féminine dans la doctrine freudienne*. Paris: Seuil.

Samama, Claude-Raphaël. (2005) "Le spirituel en psychanalyse. Images et paradigme," *Le Bloc-Notes de la Psychanalyse*, 19, pp. 111–12.

Sand, M.S., Fisher, W. et. al. (2008). "Erectile Dysfunction and Constructs of Masculinity and Quality of Life in the Multinational Men's Attitudes to Life Events and Sexuality (MALES) Study," *Journal of Sexual Medicine*, 5, pp. 583–594.

Satris, Stephen. (1995) "What Are They?" in Zack, ed.

Schindler, D.C. (2005) "Freedom Beyond Our Choosing: Augustine on the Will and Its Objects." In *Augustine and Politics*. J. Doody, K. Hughes and K. Paffenroth, eds. New York: Lexington Books.

Schofield, Malcolm. (1999) *The Stoic Idea of the City*. With a new foreword by Martha Nussbaum. Chicago: The University of Chicago Press.

Schrödinger, Erwin. (1956) *What is Life and Other Essays*. New York: Doubleday.

Searle, John R. (1995) *The Construction of Institutional Reality*. New York: The Free Press.
Shannon, Thomas A. (2005) "*Telos, Value, and Genetic Engineering*." In Harold W. Baillie and Timothy Casey, eds., *Is Human Nature Obsolete? Genetics, Bioengeneering, and the Future of the Human Condition*. Cambridge MA: MIT Press.
Sharpley-Whiting, T. Denean. (2003) "Lynching and Burning Rituals in African American Literature" in *A Companion to African-American Philosophy* Tommy L. Lott and John P. Pittmann, eds. Oxford: Blackwell.
Sheafe, Sadie M. (2007) "The Sexual Practices of Black Males and Societal Myths about Them: A Historical Overview and Contemporary Analysis," Dissertation Submitted to the Faculty of the American Academy of Clinical Sexologists in Partial Fulfillment of the Requirements for the Degree of Doctor of Philosophy (May).
Shorter, A. (2001) *African Culture: An Overview*. Nairobi: Paulines Publication.
Simmel, Georg. (1999) *Der Krieg und die geistigen Entscheidungen. Grundfragen der Soziologie. Vom Wesen des historischen Verstehens. Der Konflikt der modernen Kultur. Lebensanschauungen* (GSG 16). Frankfurt am Main: Suhrkamp.
Simon-Maeda, Andrea. (2008) "'Bigger is Better': Masculinity and Consumerist Discourses in Viagra Advertisements." In José Santaemilia and Patricia Bou, ed. *Gender and Sexual Identities in Transition*. Newcastle: Cambridge Scholars Publishing.
Sloterdijk, Peter. (1999) *Regeln für den Menschenpark*. Frankfurt am Main: Suhrkamp.
Snead, James. (1994) *White Screens, Black Images: Hollywood from the Dark Side*. New York: Routledge.
Sontag, Susan. (1969) *Styles of Radical Will*. New York: Farrar, Straus and Giroux.
Springer, Claudia. (2005) "Playing it Cool in the Matrix" in Gillis, ed.
Staehelin, Hannes B. (2005) "Promoting Health and Well-Being in Later Life." In Malcolm L. Johnson, ed. *The Cambridge Handbook of Age and Ageing*. Cambridge: Cambridge University Press.
Statman, Daniel. (1996) *Virtue Ethics*. Edinburgh: Edinburgh University Press.
Steinberger, Peter. (1996) "Who is Cephalus?," *Political Theory*, 24:2 (May), pp. 172–199.
Stieglitz, Edward J. (1949) *The Second Forty Years*. London: Staples Press.
Strauss, Leo. (1964) *City and Man*. Chicago: University of Chicago Press.
Strebhardt, Klaus and Axel Ullrich. (2008) "Paul Ehrlich's Magic Bullet Concept: 100 Years of Progress," *Nature Reviews Cancer*, 8, 473–480.
Sturgis, Frederic R. (1900) *Sexual Debility in Man*. New York: E. B. Treat & Co.
Swindle R., et al. (2004) "The Psychological and Interpersonal Relationship Scales: Assessing Psychological and Relationship Outcomes Associated with Erectile Dysfunction and Its Treatment," *Archives of Sexual Behavior*, 33:1, pp. 19–30.
Tabachnick, B.G and L.S. Fidell. (1981) *Using Multivariate Statistics*. New York: Harper and Row.
Takaki, Ronald. (1979) *Iron Cages: Race and Culture in Nineteenth-Century America*. Oxford University Press.
Tangwa, Geofrey. (2004) "Some African Reflections on Biomedical And Environmental Ethics." In Kwasi Wiredu, ed., *A Companion to African Philosophy*. Oxford: Blackwell.
thepharmaletter. (2010) "Escalating Costs of Drug Development Drive Pharmaceutical Companies to Tap Opportunities in Emerging Markets" (25 June).

http://www. thepharmaletter.com/file/ 96152/escalating-costs-of-drug-development-drive-pharmaceutical-companies-to-tap-opportunities-in-emerging-markets.html. Last accessed on 12 December 2010.

Thomson, Michael. (2008) *Endowed: Regulating the Male Sexed Body*. New York, Oxon: Routledge.

Tiefer, Leonore. (1986) "In Pursuit of the Perfect Penis: The Medicalization of Male Sexuality," *The American Behavioral Scientist* 29:5, pp. 579–600.

———. (2003) "The Pink Viagra Story: We Have the Drug but what's the Disease?" *Radical Philosophy* (September/October), 2–5, pp. 2–5.

———. (2006) "The Viagra Phenomenon," *Sexualities*, 9:3, pp. 273–294.

Toufexis, Anastasia. (1988) "It's Not All In Your Head." In *Time* (5 December): 94. http://www.time.com/time/magazine/article/0,9171,956444,00.html. Last accessed on 12 December 2010.

Traister, Bryce. (2000) "Academic Viagra: The Rise of American Masculinity Studies," *American Quarterly*, 52:2, (June), pp. 274–304.

Tropical Disease Research. (2005) *Making Health Research Work for Poor People: Progress 2003–2004*. Geneva: World Health Organization.

Trouiller, Patrice, Piero Olliaro, Els Torreele, James Orbinski, Richard Laing, and Nathan Ford. (2002) "Drug Development for Neglected Diseases: A Deficient Market and a Public-health Policy Failure," *Lancet*, 359, pp. 2188–2194.

Tuana, Nancy, ed. (2002) *Revealing Male Bodies*. Bloomington: Indiana University Press.

Valabrega, Jean-Paul. (1967) "Le problème anthropologique du fantasme." In Valabrega et al., eds., *Le désir et la perversion*. Paris: Seuil.

Vares, Tiina, and Virginia Braun. (2006) "Spreading the Word, but What Word is That? Viagra and Male Sexuality in Popular Culture," *Sexualities*, 9:3, pp. 315–332.

Vickers, J. (2009) "The Problem of Induction." http//plato.stamford.edu/archives /fall2009/entries/induction-problem/ (accessed in February 2010).

Vidyasagar, D. (2006) "Global Notes: The 10/90 Gap Disparities in Global Health Research," *Journal of Perinatology* 26:1, pp. 55–56.

Waddell, James. (1997) *Erotic Perception: Philosophical Portraits*. Lanham: University Press of America.

Wallace, Danielle M. (2007) "It's a M-A-N Thang: Black Male Gender Role Socialization and the Performance of Masculinity in Love Relationships," *The Journal of Pan African Studies*, 1:7 (March).

Weiner, Jonathan. (2010) *Long for the World*. New York: Harper Collins Ebooks.

Weischedel, Wilhelm. (1993) *Die Philosophische Hintertreppe: 34 große Philosophen in Alltag und Denken*. München: Deutscher Taschenbuch Verlag.

White, Joseph L. and James H. Cones. (1999) *Black Man Emerging: Facing the Past and Seizing the Future*. London: Routlegde.

White, Shane and Graham White. (1998) *Stylin': African American Expressive Culture from its Beginnings to the Zoot Suit*. Ithaca: Cornell University Press.

Whitehead, E. Douglas, and Terry Malloy. (1999) *Viagra: The Wonder Drug for Peak Performance*. New York: Dell Books.

WHO. (1948) "Constitution" http://www.who.int/governance/eb/constitution/en/index.html. Last accessed on 12 December 2010.

WHO. (2004) *The World Health Report 2004: Changing History*. Geneva: World Health Organization http://www.who.int/whr/2004/en/index.html. Last accessed on 12 December 2010.

William of Champeaux. (1959) *Sententiae*. In O. Lottin, ed., *Psychologie et morale au XIIe et XIIIe siècles*, Vol. V. Gembloux: Duculot.

Yoos, George E. (1985) "The Rhetoric of Cynicism," *Rhetoric Review*, 4:1, pp. 54–62.

Zack, Naomi (ed.). (1995) *American Mixed Race: The Culture of Microdiversity*. Lanham: Rowman & Littlefield.

Zack, Naomi. (1993) *Race and Mixed Race*. Philadelphia: Temple University Press.

———. (1997) "Race, Life, Identity, Tragedy, and Good Faith." In Lewis R. Gordon, ed. *Existence in Black: An Anthology of Black Existential Philosophy*. New York: Routledge.

Zemmour, Eric. (2006) *Le premier sexe*. Paris: Denoël.

Zhang, Everett Yuehong. (2007) "Switching between Traditional Chinese Medicine and Viagra: Cosmopolitanism and Medical Pluralism Today," *Medical Anthropology*, 26, pp. 53–97.

Žižek, Slavoj. (1999) *The Ticklish Subject: The Absent Center of Political Ontology*. London: Verso.

———. (2006) *The Pervert's Guide to Cinema* (Film).

General Websites:

http://www.viagra.com/about-erectile-dysfunction/erectile-dysfunction.aspx

http://media.pfizer.com/files/products/uspi_viagra.pdf.

ABOUT THE AUTHORS

THORSTEN BOTZ-BORNSTEIN was born in Germany, studied philosophy in Paris, and received his Ph.D. from Oxford University. As a postdoctoral researcher based in Finland he undertook extensive research on Russian formalism and semiotics in Russia and the Baltic countries. Since 1999 he is an Associate Researcher at the EHESS of Paris from which he received his 'habilitation.' He has also been researching in Japan, in particular on the Kyoto School and on the philosophy of Nishida Kitarô, worked for the Center of Cognition of Hangzhou University (China), and at Tuskegee University in Alabama. He is now Assistant Professor of philosophy at The Gulf University for Science and Technology in Kuwait. Publications: *Place and Dream: Japan and the Virtual* (Rodopi, 2004); *Films and Dreams: Tarkovsky, Sokurov, Bergman, Kubrik, Wong Kar-wai* (Lexington Press 2007); *Vasily Sesemann: Experience, Formalism and the Question of Being* (Rodopi 2006); *Virtual Reality: The Last Human Narrative?* (forthcoming, Rodopi 2010); *Aesthetics and Politics of Space in Russia and Japan* (Lexington 2009); *The Cool Kawaii: Afro-Japanese Aesthetics and New World Modernity* (Lexington 2010).

SOPHIE BOURGAULT is Assistant Professor at the School of Political Studies, University of Ottawa. Her main research focuses on the political thought of Plato and Jean-Jacques Rousseau, with a particular emphasis on the intersections between aesthetics, music and politics. Recent and forthcoming publications include articles in *Eighteenth-Century Thought*, the *Journal of Aesthetic Education*, *Eighteenth-Century Studies*, *Lumen*, and *1650-1850: Ideas, Aesthetics and Inquiries in the Early Modern Era*.

KEVIN GUILFOY received his Ph.D. from the University of Washington in 1997. He is currently Assistant Professor of Philosophy and coordinator of the Philosophy Politics and Economics program at Carroll University in Wisconsin. Previously, he was Assistant Professor of Philosophy at the University of Akron in Ohio. He is co-editor with Jeffery Brower of the *Cambridge Companion to Abelard* (Cambridge 2004) and has written articles on medieval logic, metaphysics and ethics. Guilfoy also writes on economic philosophy in popular culture including "Capitalism and Freedom in the Affluent Society" in *Mad Men and Philosophy* (Wiley 2010).

THOMAS KAPPER earned a doctorate that combined philosophy, law, and economics from the Gaylord Nelson Institute for Environmental Studies at the University of Wisconsin at Madison. There he was awarded the inaugural IES Landscape Research Fellowship. His dissertation was entitled, "The Economic Value of Landscape Aesthetics: Integrating Contingent Valuation and Aesthetic Assessment." He is founder and director of the firm, Peregrine Aesthetics

Group, which is concerned with the valuation of the environment and real estate. He has published articles and reviews in *Landscape Journal* and *Environmental Practice*.

ROMAN MEINHOLD is Asst. Prof. of Philosophy at the Graduate School of Philosophy & Religion, Assumption University of Thailand, Bangkok. Before working in Asia Roman taught at the National University of Lesotho, Africa and at the Weingarten University of Education, Germany. He got his MA and his Ph.D. (both Philosophy) from Johannes Gutenberg University Mainz, Germany. His areas of specialization include Philosophy of (Popular) Culture, Philosophy of Art, Applied Philosophy and Ethics. He prefers transdisciplinary approaches and is foremost interested in everyday phenomena from philosophical perspectives. His latest publications include "Popular Culture and Consumerism: Mediocre, (Schein-)Heilig, and Pseudo-Therapeutic" (in I. Yusuf & C. Atilgan (eds.) *Religion Politics and Globalization*, KAS, 2009), "Being in the Matrix: An Example of Cinematic Education in Philosophy" (*Prajna Vihara* 10/1-2, 2009), and "Black & White. On Symbolical Implications of an Aesthetical Polarization" (*Boleswa Journal of Philosophy, Theology and Religion* 1/3, 2007) amongst several others focusing on extremism & otherness, environmental issues, quality of life discourses, *eudaimonia*, and the philosophy of fashion on which also an article for the Internet Encyclopedia of Philosophy (iep.utm.edu) is in preparation. Roman also published two books on the philosophical implications fashion and lifestyle from philosophic-anthropological perspective.

ANTHONY OKEREGBE is a Lecturer in Philosophy at the University of Lagos, Lagos, Nigeria, where in 2004, he earned his Ph.D., after defending a dissertation titled "An Analysis of the Principles of Tolerance in Phenomenology." Prior to his academia career, he was a features editor of *The Guardian*, Lagos, Nigeria, with special interests on foreign affairs, religious tolerance and women lifestyle. A combination of these interests with phenomenological and existential philosophy led him to venture into researches on popular culture, public morality and leadership, areas in which he is published both locally and internationally. He is also a resource person of Lux Terrae Leadership Foundation, Nigeria, and an associate member of the Council for Research in Values and Philosophy (CRVP), Washington DC, USA.

DÓNAL O'MATHÚNA is Senior Lecturer in Ethics, Decision-Making & Evidence in the School of Nursing at Dublin City University, Ireland. He is also an academic member of the Biomedical Diagnostics Institute and the Institute of Ethics at Dublin City University. He is the author of *Nanoethics: Big Ethical Issues with Small Technology* (Continuum, 2009). He has also published articles and chapters on a variety of ethical topics, including stem cell research, human dignity, disaster research, torture, and complementary therapies. He also has a research interest in systematic reviews of the evidence for healthcare interventions and is a Visiting Fellow at the UK Cochrane Centre in Oxford, England.

CONNIE PRICE recently retired from Tuskegee University, where she taught philosophy, bioethics, and humanities for thirty-nine years. She served as Chair of the Philosophy Department for ten of those years. Her philosophical interests are contemporary continental philosophy, cinema, biopolitics, feminism, aesthetics, Bergson, Deleuze, Arendt, Langer, Kierkegaard, Nietzsche, and American pragmatism. Her doctorate in philosophy is from The Pennsylvania State University ('72). She has published several articles and participated in many organizations and research projects, at Tuskegee and on national and international bases. She continues her professional affiliations in different countries, especially Central Europe. She has also done research in Senegal. She acquired a master's degree ('88) in interactive telecommunications from New York University's Tisch School of the Arts, Graduate Institute of Film and Television. She helped create the Tuskegee University National Bioethics Center, and held a joint appointment with the Center and the Philosophy Department for her last twelve years at Tuskegee. Connie has moved to Lawrence, Kansas, where she plans to learn painting and drawing, write fiction, and continue writing about her idea ("Although they are never 'ours' alone!") of "Affective Justice."

ROBERT REDEKER, researcher at the French CNRS (Centre National de la Recherche Scientifique), is member of the editorial committee of *Les Temps modernes* and of *Des lois et des hommes*. He is also member of the scientific committee of *Quel sport?* and *Culture et droit*. He is author of: *Le Déshumain* (Toulouse: Editions Itinéraires, 2001). *Le Sport contre les peuples* (Paris: Berg, 2002), *Nouvelles figures de l'homme* (Bordeaux: Le Bord de l'eau, 2004), *Le Progrès ou l'opium de l'histoire* (Nantes: Pleins Feux, 2004), *Dépression et philosophie* (Nantes: Pleins Feux, 2007), *Le Sport est-il inhumain?* (Paris: Panama, 2008), *Egobody* (Paris: Fayard, 2010). Some of his books have been published in English by Academica Press.

BASSAM ROMAYA received his Ph.D. in philosophy from Temple University in Philadelphia. His past publications and research interest are in social and political philosophy, aesthetics, applied ethics, philosophy of sex, and GLBT Studies. His most recent publication, "The Straight Sex Experiment," appears in *College Sex and Philosophy* (in the Wiley-Blackwell Philosophy for Everyone series). He is currently Visiting Assistant Professor of Philosophy at Gettysburg College in Pennsylvania.

HERBERT ROSEMAN is an Adjunct Professor at Columbia University and St. Johns University in New York. He completed his Ph.D. at Columbia University in 2008. His dissertation was entitled *Altruism, Evolution and Optional Games*. Prior to Columbia he was a senior officer in the investment banking division of a major financial institution in New York City. He also holds a Masters degree in physics from the University of Pennsylvania and an MBA from Harvard Business School. His research interests are in the philosophy of biology especially as it relates to Darwinian evolution and it its effect on ethics. He has developed courses in behavioral economics and ethical business leadership.

CLAUDE-RAPHAËL SAMAMA received a doctorate in anthropology from the universities of Paris-Dauphine and Paris-10-Nanterre, a *diplôme d'études supérieures* (DES) in philosophy from the Sorbonne and the same diploma in clinical human sciences from the university of Paris-7. Having taught in different institutions, he is now editorial director of *L'Art du Comprendre*, a journal of history, philosophical anthropology, and hermeneutics. He is the author of many articles published in a variety of journals. His main book publications are: *Savoirs ou les jeux de l'OIR: Quantiques* (*Galilée*, 1980), *Le Livre des lunes* (Intertextes, 1992); *Les Poèmes du soi* (L'Harmattan, 1996); *Around circles. Autour des cercles,* (Caractères, 1999); *La Présence et l'exil* (L'Harmattan, 2007); *Développement mondial et culturalités. Essai d'archéologie et de prospective éco-culturales* (2001); *105 Essais de miniatures spirituelles* (2004) et *Réflexions nouvelles sur des questions juives* (2007), all published by Maisonneuve et Larose.

ROBERT VUCKOVICH is an independent scholar who earned a B.A. in Philosophy at Wilfrid Laurier University, but withdrew from a Master's program elsewhere to tend to an ailing father and then mother. He is in the process of returning to a different university to work on a thesis on Diogenes of Sinope's position on sexual practices. His areas of interest consist of stoicism, the philosophy of Fyodor Dostoevsky, sexual ethics, and rhetoric theory. He has contributed an article on deception and pedagogy to the collection, *Rhetoric, Uncertainty, and the University as Text: How Students Construct the Academic Experience* (Canadian Plains Research Center, 2007), anime and existentialism to the collection, *Everyday Fantastic: Essays on Science Fiction and Human Being* (Cambridge Scholars Publishing, 2008), and epistemological morals to the forthcoming collection *SpongeBob SquarePants and Philosophy: Soaking Up Knowledge Under the Sea* (Open Court, 2011).

INDEX

VIBS

The **Value Inquiry Book Series** is co-sponsored by:

Adler School of Professional Psychology
American Indian Philosophy Association
American Maritain Association
American Society for Value Inquiry
Association for Process Philosophy of Education
Canadian Society for Philosophical Practice
Center for Bioethics, University of Turku
Center for Professional and Applied Ethics, University of North Carolina at Charlotte
Central European Pragmatist Forum
Centre for Applied Ethics, Hong Kong Baptist University
Centre for Cultural Research, Aarhus University
Centre for Professional Ethics, University of Central Lancashire
Centre for the Study of Philosophy and Religion, University College of Cape Breton
Centro de Estudos em Filosofia Americana, Brazil
College of Education and Allied Professions, Bowling Green State University
College of Liberal Arts, Rochester Institute of Technology
Concerned Philosophers for Peace
Conference of Philosophical Societies
Department of Moral and Social Philosophy, University of Helsinki
Gannon University
Gilson Society
Haitian Studies Association
Ikeda University
Institute of Philosophy of the High Council of Scientific Research, Spain
International Academy of Philosophy of the Principality of Liechtenstein
International Association of Bioethics
International Center for the Arts, Humanities, and Value Inquiry
International Society for Universal Dialogue
Natural Law Society
Philosophical Society of Finland
Philosophy Born of Struggle Association
Philosophy Seminar, University of Mainz
Pragmatism Archive at The Oklahoma State University
R.S. Hartman Institute for Formal and Applied Axiology
Research Institute, Lakeridge Health Corporation
Russian Philosophical Society
Society for Existential Analysis
Society for Iberian and Latin-American Thought
Society for the Philosophic Study of Genocide and the Holocaust
Unit for Research in Cognitive Neuroscience, Autonomous University of Barcelona
Whitehead Research Project
Yves R. Simon Institute

Titles Published

Volumes 1 - 195 see www.rodopi.nl

196. Giuseppe Vicari, *Beyond Conceptual Dualism: Ontology of Consciousness, Mental Causation, and Holism in John R. Searle's Philosophy of Mind*. A volume in **Cognitive Science**

197. Avi Sagi, *Tradition vs. Traditionalism: Contemporary Perspectives in Jewish Thought*. Translated from Hebrew by Batya Stein. A volume in **Philosophy and Religion**

198. Randall E. Osborne and Paul Kriese, Editors, *Global Community: Global Security*. A volume in **Studies in Jurisprudence**

199. Craig Clifford, *Learned Ignorance in the Medicine Bow Mountains: A Reflection on Intellectual Prejudice*. A volume in **Lived Values: Valued Lives**

200. Mark Letteri, *Heidegger and the Question of Psychology: Zollikon and Beyond*. A volume in **Philosophy and Psychology**

201. Carmen R. Lugo-Lugo and Mary K. Bloodsworth-Lugo, Editors, *A New Kind of Containment: "The War on Terror," Race, and Sexuality*. A volume in **Philosophy of Peace**

202. Amihud Gilead, *Necessity and Truthful Fictions: Panenmentalist Observations*. A volume in **Philosophy and Psychology**

203. Fernand Vial, *The Unconscious in Philosophy, and French and European Literature: Nineteenth and Early Twentieth Century*. A volume in **Philosophy and Psychology**

204. Adam C. Scarfe, Editor, *The Adventure of Education: Process Philosophers on Learning, Teaching, and Research*. A volume in **Philosophy of Education**

205. King-Tak Ip, Editor, *Environmental Ethics: Intercultural Perspectives*. A volume in **Studies in Applied Ethics**

206. Evgenia Cherkasova, *Dostoevsky and Kant: Dialogues on Ethics*. A volume in **Social Philosophy**

207. Alexander Kremer and John Ryder, Editors, *Self and Society: Central European Pragmatist Forum*, Volume Four. A volume in **Central European Value Studies**

208. Terence O'Connell, *Dialogue on Grief and Consolation*. A volume in **Lived Values, Valued Lives**

209. Craig Hanson, *Thinking about Addiction: Hyperbolic Discounting and Responsible Agency*. A volume in **Social Philosophy**

210. Gary G. Gallopin, *Beyond Perestroika: Axiology and the New Russian Entrepreneurs*. A volume in **Hartman Institute Axiology Studies**

211. Tuija Takala, Peter Herissone-Kelly, and Søren Holm, Editors, *Cutting Through the Surface: Philosophical Approaches to Bioethics*. A volume in **Values in Bioethics**

212. Neena Schwartz: *A Lab of My Own*. A volume in **Lived Values, Valued Lives**

213. Krzysztof Piotr Skowroński, *Values and Powers: Re-reading the Philosophical Tradition of American Pragmatism*. A volume in **Central European Value Studies**

214. Matti Häyry, Tuija Takala, Peter Herissone-Kelly and Gardar Árnason, Editors, *Arguments and Analysis in Bioethics*. A volume in **Values in Bioethics**

215. Anders Nordgren, *For Our Children: The Ethics of Animal Experimentation in the Age of Genetic Engineering*. A volume in **Values in Bioethics**

216. James R. Watson, Editor, *Metacide: In the Pursuit of Excellence*. A volume in **Holocaust and Genocide Studies**

217. Andrew Fitz-Gibbon, Editor, *Positive Peace: Reflections on Peace Education, Nonviolence, and Social Change*. A volume in **Philosophy of Peace**

218. Christopher Berry Gray, *The Methodology of Maurice Hauriou: Legal, Sociological, Philosophical*. A volume in **Studies in Jurisprudence**

219. Mary K. Bloodsworth-Lugo and Carmen R. Lugo-Lugo, *Containing (Un)American Bodies: Race, Sexuality, and Post-9/11 Constructions of Citizenship*. A volume in **Philosophy of Peace**

220. Roland Faber, Brian G. Henning, Clinton Combs, Editors, *Beyond Metaphysics? Explorations in Alfred North Whitehead's Late Thought*. A volume in **Contemporary Whitehead Studies**

221. John G. McGraw, *Intimacy and Isolation (Intimacy and Aloneness: A Multi-Volume Study in Philosophical Psychology, Volume One)*, A volume in **Philosophy and Psychology**

222. Janice L. Schultz-Aldrich, Introduction and Edition, *"Truth" is a Divine Name, Hitherto Unpublished Papers of Edward A. Synan, 1918-1997*. A volume in **Gilson Studies**

223. Larry A. Hickman, Matthew Caleb Flamm, Krzysztof Piotr Skowroński and Jennifer A. Rea, Editors, *The Continuing Relevance of John Dewey: Reflections on Aesthetics, Morality, Science, and Society*. A volume in **Central European Value Studies**

224. Hugh P. McDonald, *Creative Actualization: A Meliorist Theory of Values*. A volume in **Studies in Pragmatism and Values**

225. Rob Gildert and Dennis Rothermel, Editors, *Remembrance and Reconciliation*. A volume in **Philosophy of Peace**

226. Leonidas Donskis, Editor, *Niccolò Machiavelli: History, Power, and Virtue*. A volume in **Philosophy, Literature, and Politics**

227. Sanya Osha, *Postethnophilosophy*. A volume in **Social Philosophy**

228. Rosa M. Calcaterra, Editor, *New Perspectives on Pragmatism and Analytic Philosophy*. A volume in **Studies in Pragmatism and Values**

229. Danielle Poe, Editor, *Communities of Peace: Confronting Injustice and Creating Justice*. A volume in **Philosophy of Peace**

230. Thorsten Botz-Bornstein, Editor, *The Philosophy of Viagra: Bioethical Responses to the Viagrification of the Modern World*. A volume in **Philosophy of Sex and Love**

CPSIA information can be obtained at www.ICGtesting.com
Printed in the USA
BVOW030631031011

272413BV00002B/10/P

9 789042 033368